PENGUIN BOOKS

tell me the truth

Dr Ranjana Srivastava was educated in India, the United Kingdom, the United States and Australia. She graduated from Monash University with a first-class honours degree and several awards in medicine. In 2004 she won the prestigious Fulbright Award, which she completed at the University of Chicago. Ranjana is now an oncologist and educator in the Melbourne public hospital system.

Ranjana's writing has been featured in *Time, The Week, New York Times, The Age* and *Best Australian Science Writing,* and in numerous medical journals including the *New England Journal of Medicine* and *The Lancet.* In 2008 her story 'Ode to a Patient' won the Cancer Council Victoria Arts Award for outstanding writing and in 2012 Ranjana won the Gustav Nossal Prize for Global Health writing. She has published two books: *Tell Me the Truth,* which was shortlisted for the NSW Premier's Literary Award, and the warmly received Penguin Special *Dying for a Chat,* which addresses the lack of communication between doctors and patients.

Ranjana lives in Melbourne with her husband and three young children.

tell me the truth

Conversations with my patients about life and death

DR RANJANA SRIVASTAVA

PENGUIN BOOKS

PENGUIN BOOKS

UK | USA | Canada | Ireland | Australia
India | New Zealand | South Africa | China

Penguin Books is part of the Penguin Random House group of companies
whose addresses can be found at global.penguinrandomhouse.com.

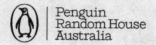
Penguin
Random House
Australia

First published by Penguin Group (Australia), 2010
This edition published by Penguin Group (Australia), 2014

Cover design by Deb Billson © Penguin Group (Australia)
Text design by Kirby Armstrong © Penguin Group (Australia)
Cover image © Photolibrary
Typeset in Fairfield Light by Sunset Digital Publishing Services, Brisbane, Queensland
Printed and bound in Australia by Griffin Press, an accredited ISO AS/NZS 14001
Environmental Management Systems printer.

National Library of Australia
Cataloguing-in-Publication data:

Srivastava, Ranjana.
Tell me the truth: conversations with my patients
about life and death / Ranjana Srivastava
9780143571148 (paperback)
Physician and patient. Communication in medicine.
Cancer–Patients–Attitudes.

362.196994

penguin.com.au

To
my parents, Urmila and Kaushal,
and my brother, Rajesh,
for always believing

Contents

The truth is rarely pure and never simple.

— Oscar Wilde, *The Importance of Being Earnest*

I

◇

Lessons from my Nanima

Few doctors stumble into becoming a cancer specialist. My earliest brush with the disease came when I was ten and my beloved grandmother, my Nanima, was diagnosed with the disease at a late stage. She went from a healthy and devout woman to a vulnerable and ailing patient, all within a period of weeks. Her transformation was as devastating as it was complete. Although I was young, there were many occasions during the last phase of her life that left an impression on me. It is only as I grew older and became a doctor that these memories, once isolated episodes, formed the scaffolding of the realisation that the same issues that had affected my Nanima still haunted the lives of modern cancer patients.

Back then, numbed by sadness, my family had assumed that the technology, especially in provincial India, simply wasn't there to save her or help us come to terms with her demise. But how was it that, when medical science had advanced beyond our wildest imagination – even treating diseases that were once deemed incurable – many patients and families still echoed the sentiments we felt all those years ago? Could it be that, infatuated by the science of medicine, we had ignored its art?

I became an oncologist to find out for myself but also to be a part of the remedy. I quickly discovered, to my disappointment, that patients like my Nanima existed everywhere. They were everyday people – somebody's parent, somebody's child, a grandmother or a husband. One day they felt well, another day something just did not seem right. It took weeks, maybe months, to diagnose the condition, and when the diagnosis was made, it was one whose very name filled the mind with a sense of unfathomable foreboding and unending sorrow. The betrayal of the body continued when it defied treatment, or when it played along initially, only to succumb without warning to the ravages of cancer.

Tracking the progress of patients, I saw, unbelievingly at first, that what my family had witnessed then was far from an anachronism today. My Nanima, long hospitalised, had scant contact with her oncologist. Her husband didn't even find out her diagnosis until well into her disease and her children fed hungrily on the infrequent morsels of information relayed through her eldest son, who, despite being highly educated, struggled to gain a clear picture of the situation. So it was that we all drifted in the fog of misconception and breathed in an air of desperate, but ultimately false, hope until my Nanima sank into a coma and died.

The oncologist who treated my Nanima came highly recommended and no doubt applied all the available knowledge in treating her. But twenty-five years on from her death, our grief sometimes still seems palpable and unresolved. I wish that the oncologist had held my Nanima's hand and told her what to expect. I know that she, being the devout woman she was, would have chosen to go home to die, and pray at the same temple where she prayed for a happy marriage, healthy children and many grandchildren. I wish the oncologist had told us that although my Nanima's death was inevitable, our aimless walks through perpetual corridors of fear and guilt were not. I wish he had made the time to talk to us and answer the questions that tortured our minds. Why did she get cancer? Was she in pain? How much longer did she have to suffer?

Cancer patients, and indeed sufferers of a multitude of other terminal illnesses and their loved ones, face the same conundrums and express many of the same misgivings today. I know now that there are still no sophisticated answers to these questions. But what I also see is that even after twenty-five years of trying, it can be hard to fully reconcile with a death that was not accompanied by the treating doctor's compassion, honesty and sensitivity.

My family's experiences were not unique then and would not be so now. As I treat my own patients, I find plenty of gaps in the care they receive from me and my colleagues. Official reports abound with the factual errors doctors make, such as operating on the wrong side of the body or prescribing the incorrect drug, but what they do not register are the more frequent, everyday occasions when we do not talk to our patients as fully as we ought or when we fail to address their concerns that we know lurk beneath the surface – sometimes because we lack the time, but often because we are unsure how to do so.

The patients in this book were once ordinary people going about their day-to-day lives. They were parents, grandparents, carers, accountants, doctors and lawyers. Something about their cancer journey left an impression on me, whether it was frustration at my inability to effectively combat their disease or my hesitation, ill-calculated, in engaging in a timely and meaningful conversation with them and their families. Within these pages, there are patients who beat the odds and returned triumphantly, and others who desperately made me wish that they too could have lived longer because their very presence served to enrich humanity. There are stories of moral conflict, ethical dilemmas and squandered opportunity. Ten years on from when I had my first taste of oncology as a junior doctor, there is an overdue reflection on how the experience changed my life. Some years after qualifying as an oncologist, I would also learn how no amount of professional loss prepares one for the intrusion of a personal tragedy. Just when I thought I understood the essentials of being an oncologist, I became a mother. I had expected motherhood to transform the landscape of my personal life but I had never imagined the enormous impact it would have on my relationship with my patients. Suddenly, heartaches were magnified, priorities altered. I found myself at one with parents who cared more to go home and spend their last days at the beach with their children than have another round of chemotherapy.

There is an undercurrent of sadness to many of my encounters, but I see them as stories that salute the remarkable human spirit. Every individual's battle with cancer and every family's ordeal in the process is somewhat different. But the longer I practise, the more I discover how courageously cancer patients take on a challenge they did not ever bargain for. These patients do not see themselves as valiant or tenacious; indeed, among other things, cancer erodes self-confidence so much that many openly feel unremarkable and ordinary. I hope my recollections prove that their sentiments are a far cry from the truth, for I find my patients nothing short of inspiring. Their perspective is hard-won but invaluable. Despite the scourge of illness, they somehow bear the grace and resilience of many. And their courage in facing up to life's inevitable but greatest blow is as remarkable as it is hard to truly fathom.

Being a doctor, especially an oncologist, allowed into the most intimate recesses of patients' lives, is an extraordinary privilege. The experiences – humbling, levelling and thought-provoking – have long been my companion; a private well of strength and succour.

Every patient provides a lesson in the long road to becoming a better doctor, a more complete oncologist. In a corner of my heart, I cannot help but feel that heeding these lessons, sharing them, and using them in the days that lie ahead, is the best tribute that I can pay my beloved Nanima.

2

◇

I feel better for having met you

The year was 1999. My year-long internship was over, the pathos and drama of an intense and enjoyable year barely covered by a certificate that blandly confirmed I had fulfilled all the requirements to move from provisional to full registration as a medical practitioner.

Now, I was spoilt for and bewildered by choices. I could choose to leave the hospital setting and become a general practitioner in the community, but I was attracted to the collegiality, intellect and patient mix of the hospital setting. Positive supervisor reports had also opened the doors to literally any speciality of my choosing. I knew surgery was not for me, underlined by the surgeons' complete disdain at my two episodes of fainting at the sight of a human body laid open. But anaesthetics sounded inviting, especially when the consultant sold the lifestyle so well: family friendly, flexible and lucrative. He talked about skiing mid-week and spending vacations with his kids. I didn't have any children but I saw them in my future; having holidays with them sounded both normal and welcome. Then the director of the emergency department called: 'We would love you to join us. Try us out, I think you will thrive here.'

Just two years earlier, I was an unknown medical student, wandering around the same emergency department, searching for any doctor who would teach me something. Now, its director had come calling with a job. It sounded too good to be true.

I flirted with psychiatry until my parents groaned – only half-jokingly, I suspected – 'Why don't you become a real doctor?'

In turn, I attended interviews with the heads of dermatology and pathology. One lured me with the low-stress, family-friendly, high-paying lifestyle, the other with the still memorably deadpan statement, 'At least your patients will never talk back to you.'

My childhood friend in India, having herself entered paediatrics training, watched me with growing bemusement. 'I don't believe it,' she finally said. 'You know you are a physician at heart.'

So, with a troubled mind I applied to become a specialist physician, unable to reconcile with taking sole responsibility for settling on a career. At my interview with a senior physician, who was a cardiologist, I feigned an enthusiasm proportional to my anxiety, which only grew as the welcoming offer arrived. I enviously regarded those colleagues who seemed utterly confident in their choice of speciality.

I was unlucky enough to spend my first three months of physician training doing night shifts. After this desultory term, where I did not see or hear anything even remotely affirming, I was sent to a rural hospital to do oncology. At the time, being sent on a rural rotation was akin to exile, even a temporary absence from the nerve centre of one's primary or parent hospital signalling a doomed career. 'No one of importance gets to know you', I heard someone complain. My misgivings compounded, I set off on my three-month adventure, resigned to my fate.

On my first day, I had to wait until eight p.m. to do a ward round. The second ward round ran later and the third even more so.

Devouring a bowl of cold pasta from the cafeteria, I naively concluded that my boss was either very slow or very thorough. But it didn't take me long to realise that, late as they were, and conducted between silent yawns, the rounds were becoming the scintillating focus of my long days. Through corridors that had long fallen silent in the wake of chatty visitors and rattling meal trolleys, the oncologist and I walked from room to room, reviewing some of the sickest patients in the hospital, breaking bad news, discussing treatment and complications, even chatting at length with the odd family member who had stayed back to catch us. He stood ready to demystify cancer to both his patients and an equally nonplussed, fresh resident who sometimes embarrassingly needed to look up the long names of drugs. The oncologist seemed equally at ease switching gears and discussing the fortunes of a football team or the latest global political crisis with a keen patient. The rounds were interesting, as much for the medicine they taught me as for the other lessons that were so subtle I could have dismissed them, had I not been in a reflective frame of mind about my career and desperate to figure out what made other people stick to theirs.

One night we met a fit forty-year-old woman and a shrunken old man from a nursing home, both suffering from an aggressive lymphoma. One was lined up for intensive curative treatment, and the other for palliation. We spent an equal amount of time with both but discussed very different matters. With one, the oncologist spoke about the physical and emotional rigours of chemotherapy but the reasonable long-term prognosis; with the other, he dwelt on the importance of pain management, comfort care and time spent with family. But he showed equal concern for his judgement regarding both. The old man, wasting rapidly and huddled under bedcovers that weighed him down, was too frail to ask questions, but it didn't prevent the oncologist from visiting him every single night, no matter how late, until the day he died. I reassured him on the especially late nights that our patients were stable and could wait to be seen the next evening, but no matter how late it was, we would go on a round. I could not help but notice that even when the old man lost the capacity to talk, his eyes responded to the oncologist's presence. I found the routine comforting but also inspiring. This was my first realisation that the same cancer comes with different scripts for different patients and that caring was as important as curing.

I made many mistakes during the rotation. They were mainly borne of inexperience, such as assessing pain incompletely, being too hasty in providing reassurance without understanding the full extent of disease, or doing a blood test too few or too many. My mistakes frustrated me and sowed seeds of doubt in my mind about my adequacy, but I never went to sleep feeling like this, because on our rounds, the oncologist corrected the misinformation and misconception, with no fuss and much goodwill, leaving my uncertainties to dissipate and me to face another day of treating his patients with renewed enthusiasm. I never became enamoured of the long hours but I fell in love with my job and recognised clearly the crucial importance of chancing upon a good mentor.

However, even as many weeks went by, I could never bring myself to see the oncologist's patients as anything but his. It was as if, despite carrying both our names on the handover sheets, there was an invisible plaque over every bed that proclaimed the patient's strict ownership. The oncologist trusted me but I couldn't trust myself with his patients, who seemed to have such a tight relationship with their oncologist. I kept wondering how and why.

One morning, I was asked to see a lady who had been admitted overnight. Jane was in her fifties, a pleasant woman, obviously ravaged by breast cancer. She had come in severely short of breath due to the accumulation of fluid in her lung. Three litres were drained overnight and she reported feeling much better, although it was clear that her respiration was still laboured. The new onset of back pain sounded an ominous warning in the face of chemotherapy. I found her easy to deal with because she seemed outwardly calm and composed, which must have been difficult for one in her precarious position. I checked that her oxygen levels were adequate and increased her painkillers. I talked to the radiation doctors about treating her back pain and arranged an urgent scan. I knew that her husband had a sudden business trip and her children lived far away, so I asked a volunteer to drop by and keep her company. I felt sad that her prognosis was poor but felt it beyond my capability or brief to discuss her future. But I saw her three times that day to ensure her comfort. By evening, she acknowledged that her breathing felt even better and the painkillers I had prescribed were taking effect.

Our ward round that night was particularly long. We passed Jane's room and I heard her stir inside then settle back as she saw that we had moved on. But we finally returned to her door. The oncologist murmured that he had a headache and was glad this was the last patient.

'She looks fairly comfortable now so this shouldn't take long,' I added, also keen to see him finish his unimaginably long day and week. I remember looking at my watch as my boss entered. It was ten p.m. Jane's dark single room was illuminated only by a dim light which made it impossible to make out anything much. I hung back a step, to wait for the nurse to get her chart.

From my place at the door, I saw her shadow jump up in bed. Jane's first words to her oncologist were almost shouted with relief: 'I feel better just knowing you are here!'

Such was the radiant warmth and complete trust in her voice

that I instinctively held back. But two things struck me immediately. I had spent the better half of my day weaving in and out of her room and she had expressed her gratitude graciously enough, but the greeting she had reserved for her oncologist was of an entirely different nature. She had welcomed my intervention but was celebrating his mere presence at her bedside. Perhaps she had feared he wouldn't come, but I knew that her tearful words expressed more than relief – they were a ringing declaration of her unyielding faith in him. Simple words that they were, they announced that even though she knew her life was imperilled, her immediate welfare was guaranteed now that he had arrived.

My second concurrent realisation was that in my several years of medical training thus far, I had never before witnessed anything like this. As a surgical intern, I had seen plenty of patients in awe of the surgeon who had removed their bleeding ulcer or salvaged their gangrenous foot. When the surgeon came by, they would regard him with veneration, too dumbstruck for words at this living incarnation of divinity who had cupped their life in his hands. 'Thank you for saving his life,' a trembling wife would mouth. On the medical unit, the heroics were more subtle, accordingly acknowledged by the occasional note or box of chocolates. 'Thank you for all your help and care,' the note would say. But not even once in all those years had I seen a patient express such profound relief at the mere sight of their doctor, as if this doctor and this doctor alone held their confidence.

After nearly half an hour, the oncologist emerged from Jane's room.

'Sorry, I thought you had left. You should have come in.'

I didn't say that I had spent the time wondering how one earns such extraordinary loyalty from patients, how a doctor transcends the divide between being respected and being actually cherished.

'Was she okay?'

'Yes. You did all the right things. Thank you.'

Then why is it that she still felt better for seeing you? I wanted to ask without sounding churlish. I surprised even myself to discover that I did not feel slighted by the experience, only lifted.

If ever there was an inspired moment in my professional life, it was this. I knew it then and I can see it just as clearly now. I knew that I wanted to be an oncologist, but not just any oncologist; I wanted to be like the one I had witnessed that night. After that, I never once looked back in doubt.

More than ten years on from that singular experience, I now return to the same rural hospital by choice, to relieve that same oncologist when he takes the occasional break. I find the respect and affection that he commanded then only magnified with the passage of time. Even though I am now in a more qualified position to help his patients, it is as clear to me today as it was then that their bond with him was not something my insecure mind had concocted.

Much in my life has changed since the days when I was an uncertain and reluctant resident banished to the country. I am now an oncologist, a wife and a mother to three delightful children, including a newborn. My life suddenly seems fuller than I had ever predicted.

I also have patients of my own. And my proudest and most humbling moments in medicine come when my patients say what I had never imagined I would hear: 'I feel better for having seen you.' This, to me, is the highest accolade a patient can pay a doctor. These are the words that convert my work from a job to a vocation.

'But isn't it depressing?' I am frequently asked, by doctors and non-doctors alike.

To this I say no. It may be depressing on the surface but caring for cancer patients is ultimately a deeply humanising and levelling experience. My clinics are filled with patients who led ordinary and largely content lives before being rudely thrown into the vortex of a cancer diagnosis. But they are transformed by their diagnosis into extraordinary individuals who amaze us all.

'There's nothing amazing about me,' the patient sighs wearily. 'I am just doing what I need to do.'

But it *is* amazing what patients do. They dig deep within themselves to find resilience they never knew they had; they reignite sometimes painful relationships to give them their due justice; they coach their damaged bodies to live with the ravages of cancer; they bend their minds to accept the inevitable end. Others wake up every day to make the winding drive to chemotherapy, endure long and nauseating waits in cramped rooms, shrug off the vagaries of the hospital bureaucracy, and appreciate their carers even when the care is failing. Cancer patients put up with the most and complain the least, endowed with an uncommon wisdom that is a privilege to observe. It is not simply that they see the big picture; if you spend long enough with them, they help you see it too.

On a superficial level, you realise that traffic jams and long queues are not worth sweating over. Neither are hostile people or vexatious relationships. You are grateful that the fatigue in your muscles is only the result of a long run. Or that your symptoms amount to nothing more than a common cold.

But on a deeper level, you learn that you cannot overstate the importance of family, love and close relationships in life. Or the gratification of spending a little more time simply enjoying your children, minus the hidden agenda of shaping their whole lives. You learn the value of having a sanctum within your soul that you can access when all around you there is turbulence. And of cultivating throughout your life an inner peace so that when the end is near, you can look back at a lifetime and not feel harassed by regrets.

Once upon a time they sounded like lofty ideals, but being an oncologist has placed me firmly in their touch and sight. I appreciate what my patients unwittingly teach me. I like and respect the way they help me grow, not only as a doctor, but also as a daughter, mother and wife.

Sometimes I think it would not be too late to start saying to my patients, 'I feel better for having met you.'

3

◇

Find the will to start

Following a short drive, I sidestep shards of broken glass and used syringes to cross to the refugee centre, which is located in a cheaply rented house in a drug-addled part of town. The snoopy parking inspector marks my car, taking perverse delight in handing out the fines I regularly incur. Once I protested that I was always running late because it takes longer than expected to sort through a room full of non-English-speaking people who are even less able to communicate because they are unwell.

'Tell that to the council!' he smirked.

I walk up the creaking stairs to the sparsely furnished reception. A collection of ageing couches is scattered around the small area. The foam stuffing from one is coming apart and another seems too sunken to risk sitting down in. There is a roughly drawn sign that requests volunteers to drive refugee families to an upcoming picnic, which threatens to be cancelled if not enough drivers are found. A set of postcards bears the face of a sleeping baby in mandatory detention. The sign above the infant exhorts volunteers to send a postcard to the government to protest keeping children in detention. A group of young Afghan refugees huddles in a corner, waiting patiently to consult the volunteer legal team that will help process its migration application.

I unlock the tiny room that serves as my office and the pharmacy. Out-of-date books crowd a tired-looking wooden desk, atop which sits a worn blood-pressure monitor. Lately I have been afraid of using it lest the cuff split open. Two mismatched chairs, a thin, hard examination bed, and a cupboard, rapidly emptying of its donated contents, fill the rest of the room. It is a far cry from the well-appointed consulting suites of the hospital whose premises I have just left. I scan the messages and unchecked reports that have accumulated in the last week, grateful there is nothing that should have been addressed earlier. This clinic is conducted by a skeleton staff of doctors who get by on borrowed hours, hope and luck. It is a tribute to the human body that patients largely get better and avoid bad outcomes.

My first patient is a man in his fifties. He nods pleasantly, thanking me for my time.

'Doctor, would you please check my blood pressure?' He speaks fluent English with a beautiful lilt.

'Of course,' I reply, sneaking a warning look at the ailing instrument. As I coax the squeaky cuff into action, I make conversation. I learn that he was a prominent lawyer in his home country who spent his life fighting cases on behalf of his ordinary fellow citizens. Then disaster struck. The government came after him, his family was persecuted, and he lost his job. His wife left him, considering him a prime target for assassination and, in search of a better life for his children, he fled his war-torn nation to seek asylum. Now he is in limbo, classified as an illegal immigrant while he awaits a pronouncement on his appeal to be accepted as a refugee. Draconian as his journey sounds, it is not unusual for his countrymen. I hear similar stories every week. I sense there is more to come.

'Where are your children?'

'In a small village, hiding with relatives.'

'Do you speak with them?'

'Rarely, when they travel to the city to use a payphone.'

I am discomfited by his palpable grief.

'You remind me of my children,' he says. 'One day, they had a future like yours. Now they are lucky to be alive.'

'What do you do all day?' I continue, not knowing how to agree.

'I look for employment. I will be a clerk in a back room somewhere. I don't mind. Anything I can do to forget this madness.'

The toning down of his aspirations does not go unnoticed by me.

'Do you have a place to stay?'

'The Red Cross shelter. Thank goodness for the Red Cross. I spent a few nights on the cold streets before some people referred me to this centre. They linked me up with the Red Cross.'

His tears now flow freely at his shameful predicament. He makes no effort to wipe them away. Like a cascade, his words tumble out, starting from when he began his career to when he gained prominence, to his marriage and divorce. Interspersed are hints of the violence in his country and the day-to-day danger of living that forced him away to an unexpected existence of even greater uncertainty. His allotted half-hour passes without either of us rising. He needs to tell his story; I am compelled to listen. He dissolves once again into tears, collects himself, then cries again. I feel myself swimming alongside him in a sea of helplessness. I am sorry and ashamed at his plight. Forty-five minutes later, he is exhausted.

'Thank you, doctor. I have not spoken freely to anybody for five months.'

As a non sequitur I offer to resume checking his blood pressure.

It is high and I hand him appropriate medication. He accepts the pills with some hesitation.

'What will happen when they run out?'

'I will renew your supply,' I reassure him, praying that a month's reprieve to find some drug donations will be adequate.

My next question catches him unaware. 'Are you hungry?'

The denial comes quickly. 'Oh no, I'm fine!'

'Have lunch anyway. The volunteers have made some.'

He averts his eyes.

Next is a primary school teacher in her twenties. She stares mutely at me for several minutes. Bewildered and concerned, I go through a normal history-taking process with her, hoping that something will emerge. Without explanation, she draws both hands over her ears and looks straight out the window. I don't know what to do, so I wait. Then, slowly, stumblingly, over the next hour she unfolds the account of her repeated rape by rebel militia in her home country and her barefoot escape through thick jungles with packs of soldiers in pursuit. The details are intentionally patchy, but her visible fear and continuing trauma are overpowering. Thousands of miles away, I shudder with her as she sketches an image of barbed wire, forced imprisonment, fleeing from the sound of guns and daily nightmares that are so real she can touch them. I feel sickness rising within me, helpless and so completely out of my depth. Nothing in my medical training has prepared me for dealing with such tragedy. I want to ask her to stop, horrified at what fellow human beings are capable of. But how can I muzzle her courageous revelations to prevent my own discomfort? Fortunately, she herself stops, overcome by emotion.

I know that she needs urgent and qualified help.

'Would you like to speak with someone who could help you a little more?'

'No, I just want to die.'

There is no female counsellor on our books, even if I could convince the patient to recount her horror.

'You have come through so much and now you are safe. Please let us try to help you.'

'Only death will scrub my shame.'

I am concerned about her risk of suicide. If she were a documented resident of this country, there would be some avenues of urgent support for her, including involuntary admission to a psychiatric hospital. But she is illegal and beyond the realm of such care. She leaves the room and I let her leave. It is one of the most unethical and heart-wrenching decisions I will make. A few days later, I discover that the stress of her illegal status compounded by the ignominy of her ordeal has driven her to flee this country too. I never managed to keep my promise of calling her again so we could talk some more.

In quick succession, I see an Afghan woman with dandruff who has looked everywhere to find a female physician, an elderly East Timorese man with poorly controlled asthma and a Burmese student who has persistent migraines after being released from detention. He escaped across the border after months of planning and has regretted the decision ever since. He is young and misses his parents, not realising that the practical difficulties of finding food and shelter could be insurmountable. He has experienced depressive symptoms for months. His dark eyes are dull with the drudgery of life and I cannot find a single item in his life to relate to. Then I mention the Burmese leader under house arrest, Aung San Suu Kyi, observing that she is a graceful and courageous woman. His eyes light up in agreement as well as wide-eyed wonder that someone is even vaguely familiar with his beloved country. This is the opening I need to talk to him about depression.

A terminally ill Lebanese man, living alone, wants a letter for the immigration minister, to allow his only son to visit him. The man's wife died during a protracted migration approval process. His son has previously been refused entry to the country on security grounds. In the past few months, the man's prostate cancer has spread widely.

'Doctor, I can't come back to see you too often,' he say softly. 'Someone has to carry me up and down the stairs every time.' He lives upstairs, in a small, basic one-room lodge provided by the Red Cross. The wives of some of his countrymen bring him food and the men do his shopping, but everyone works and he has become increasingly dependent on their goodwill for the arrangement to continue. He desperately wishes for his son to join him in the twilight of his life.

'Young men from Lebanon can sometimes just be sons, doctor,' he remarks, a subtle reference to widely reported concerns about terrorism.

I pen a letter of support to the Department of Immigration, confident it will fail. The sheet of paper I hand him is embossed neither with the imprimatur of a hospital nor a significant individual. I tell him plainly that I am afraid my plea will mean little to the authorities, although it weighs heavily on my heart.

'Thank you for trying, at least.'

I cannot help but note that in the months I have known him, we have never even touched on the matter of treating his cancer. In my parallel world of cancer at the hospital, I would present him with several options, none of which would eradicate his cancer, but would go a long way towards managing his pain and delaying complications. But idealistic as I may be accused of being, I too recognise my limits. Despite being an educated man, he never once asks me about treatment either. It is as if, in assuming that his untreated cancer is his cross to bear alone, he wants to spare us both the discomfort of confronting the awkward truth.

'Is there anything else I can do for you, Mr Al-Abaid?'

He hesitates.

'What is it?'

'My pain. But I don't have too much money —'

'I know, I know.' I cut him off. I hate hearing about the penury of refugee patients and sometimes retreat into my own denial when there is nothing I can do. When you claim to be a refugee, with the onus of proof on your shoulders, should you also have to prove that your pain is authentic?

'You shouldn't have to be in pain,' I decide aloud for him.

'This is my fate, doctor.' He says this without a hint of censure or self-pity.

I call the palliative care physician at my hospital. Working closely with him, I have come to notice his open-heartedness in dealing with the dying. He tells me that his community palliative care team shoulders the responsibility of tending to dying refugees without delving into their past.

'He can't pay for any drugs,' I warn the physician. 'And he is going to need morphine.'

'We will figure something out.' They are the most lavish words I have heard all day.

Relieved, I explain to Mr Al-Abaid that specialised nurses will make contact with him to manage his pain and provide some emotional support during this difficult time. I also warn him that as he is a charitable case, he may not receive too many visits.

'I am afraid this is not much,' I apologise, thinking that what I would say to a similar patient in the hospital setting would be, 'I can reassure you that we have many ways of treating your pain.'

'It will just be good to see a friendly face,' he says, bowing deeply at the unforeseen aid.

The still, oppressive heat of the afternoon seems to magnify the queue of waiting patients. A young woman separates herself from the crowd.

'Excuse me, doctor, how long will you be?'

I answer with a flicker of annoyance, 'I am not sure but I *will* see you.'

An hour later it is her turn. She looks far too well, I silently judge. The well-worried, a term doctors use for those who just think they are sick. She springs from her seat at the sound of her name but moves away from me towards the stairs. There, she utters a rapid command in a foreign tongue before turning apologetically towards me. Before I can greet her, a scarf-clad head comes into view. It belongs to an elderly woman supported, almost dragged, up the stairs by two solid-looking men. The men stop on the landing, then wordlessly and cautiously lift her up into the air and carry her to the chair in my room. Her features are wizened, her frame shrunken beyond the six decades stated on her chart. Her eyes are dull, opaque; her face a repository of apprehension, anxiety, perhaps much more. She periodically glances at her daughter but mostly she keeps her face averted as we settle into the consultation. Familiar with this style of consultation, especially at the refugee clinic where patients have a limited grasp of language and culture, I let the daughter speak for her mother.

'I am sorry if I was rude, doctor. My mother has cancer and she was waiting downstairs for a long time. My family is here legally but she is considered a refugee. We don't have the money to see a private specialist. Someone told me that you may be able to help.'

I am caught unaware. This is a refugee clinic, run out of a makeshift set-up as bare as any in the Third World. Volunteer physicians bring their own equipment and, often, the spare drug samples we hand out. Limited doctors and meagre donations mean we can barely treat hypertension, eczema and headaches, and are rarely able to provide refugees with anything remotely resembling the standard of care taken for granted in the wider community.

'We don't *do* cancer,' I want to say, keen to end the conversation right there. Mr Al-Abaid is in reception, sitting in a corner, waiting to be carried home. 'Just ask him,' I feel like adding. 'He knows.'

'My mother needs a doctor. They said *you* would help.' Her voice is a mix of pleading, frustration and accusation. The mother winces with pain. The daughter solicitously measures out some morphine. As the patient swallows it with a wry face, her daughter murmurs, 'This is the last morphine. We have to wait now until . . .'

'Until . . .?'

She shakes her head. I completely miss the warning.

'Until what?'

'Until my husband's disability pension arrives.'

She runs a brusque hand across the involuntary tears that have started. Her mother's hand surreptitiously reaches out from under the folds of her dress to comfort her daughter. The mother does not need to speak English to understand the exchange that has just occurred. I know because she slowly lifts her face to me, her eyes full of reproach. In that moment the enormity and heartache of the situation descends on me and Mrs Habib becomes my patient.

'My mother probably had the cancer for many months but didn't want to trouble me. It is only when I noticed blood on her blouse that I found out.' She took her mother to her own general practitioner who used her connections to obtain a surgical appointment. The surgeon was able to arrange a free mastectomy at a public hospital on compassionate grounds.

'The surgeon saw us once afterwards, said the scar had healed and that his job was done. We were told an oncologist would take over her care.'

'Was an appointment made for you to see one?'

'No. I tried myself but was told that refugees like my mum could not get an appointment.'

'Did anyone else help you?'

'No.'

It is a familiar theme.

'So tell me what happened next.'

'We went to a private oncologist.' She sneaks a glance at her mother. 'Maybe you can read the letters.' This time, I note the subtle change of tone in her voice, urging me to be sensitive.

I read two letters from the oncologist, noting her inability to pay and his to continue her care. A further such letter from a second oncologist marks a trail of disappointment.

'The oncologist gave us a few sample pills,' she remarks, before adding what she really wants to say: 'and then said it was a good pill and she needed five years of it.' She visibly smarts at the recommendation that proved to be a mere tantalisation for her, as she could not afford to keep her mother on the drug.

'So what's the last thing you were told about the cancer?'

'Our local doctor says that her pain means it has spread to the bones.'

I feel burdened by the realisation of my undertaking. How will I adequately treat or even determine the true extent of her cancer? Where will her drugs come from? Who will do her blood tests? What will happen when she becomes terminally ill? The near-empty drug cupboard stares at me insolently. Reminders of battles past to achieve a modicum of care for far less sick refugees fill with me foreboding. Distracting myself from the panic, I state aloud, 'First we need to control your pain. Then we can think about all the other things.'

Although cancer patients describe a dizzying array of intolerable symptoms, two that disproportionately distress me are pain and vomiting. Troubles such as nausea, anxiety or insomnia are intangible, and hence unfairly subject to rationalisation on the part of doctors. 'Of course, I would be anxious too if this were happening to me,' I have remarked on more than one occasion. But there is no ignoring the sudden lightning rod of pain that pierces the patient's body, causing it to stiffen in surprise, stalling conversation. There is no denying the reflexive wince when no posture is comfortable, no intervention successful. Similarly, vomiting has always seemed to me a stark visual demonstration of how cancer and chemotherapy exact revenge on a broken body. I hate witnessing the helplessness with which a patient must surrender to the errant body, for the waves of vomiting will recede when they will. There is no soothing hand or emollient word that will quell the demon before its time.

Mrs Habib is clearly distressed with her pain as she shifts unobtrusively in her chair. I wonder if the sensation of pain is heightened when you know that treatment has run out. Or does this very fact raise the threshold for experiencing pain? I shudder to think that Mrs Habib could be the unwitting experimental case for this unsavoury question.

At my request, the clinic nurse locates a disused pack of donated morphine. When she comes in with the drug, she mentions in an aside to me that after making extensive phone calls, she has located a pharmacist willing to supply Mrs Habib's cancer pill, Tamoxifen, at cost price. Tamoxifen is one of the oldest, cheapest, yet most effective drugs for breast cancer. It is usually well-tolerated and does not need the same rigorous observation for side effects that many other therapies require. I congratulate the nurse on her find.

Mrs Habib still has the original Tamoxifen script that she was never able to afford and I now take it from her daughter. The nurse kindly reassures the daughter that the clinic will do everything it can to ensure Mrs Habib's comfort. I force myself to smile encouragingly, telling myself that we will succeed.

At a sign from the daughter, the two men come inside, swing Mrs Habib into their arms and carry her down to the waiting car. The daughter hangs back.

'How long does she have, doctor? She looks so sick . . .'

'Without knowing the true extent of her disease, I can't really say.' For once, I want to say, I really mean it, I am not being circumspect.

Fresh tears fall from her eyes. 'Can you see what it's like not knowing?'

I nod mutely, troubled by her grief and my growing concern.

From then on, Mrs Habib's care occupies most of my weekly slot at the refugee clinic. I set aside an hour to deal with her needs and try to get through the other patients as swiftly as possible, praying that I do not uncover any pressing needs in their health. When she returns after a week, she has used up almost all of the liquid morphine.

'I am sorry,' says her daughter tersely, 'but she is in a lot of pain.'

'You don't have to justify your use of morphine,' I reply, conscious of how unthinkingly this drug and others are wasted in the hospital when only a fraction of a vial is used and the rest casually discarded.

For the first time in my career, I set about trying to obtain routine tests on a non-routine patient. I start with my hospital. I call the radiology department to order a CT scan to determine the extent of Mrs Habib's cancer.

'What's her unit record number?' asks the secretary.

'She doesn't have one.'

'Okay, then her Medicare number will do.'

'She doesn't have one of those either.'

'Then I can't accept her booking. Who is this person anyway?'

I cannot help but notice that out of the six people I plead my case to, not one comments on the obvious plight of my patient. I think about appealing to my own boss, but after an earlier exchange still burning in my mind, I feel hopeless.

The daughter watches silently as I hang up the phone in frustration.

'I will figure out a way to get a scan,' I say, 'but it might just take some time.'

'Sure, doctor.'

The next time the men carry Mrs Habib in, she looks wan. She has had severe headaches for the past three days, now accompanied by vomiting. Her head sits poised over a plastic bag the whole time she is there.

'My husband's friend let us have two of his sleeping pills,' her daughter says, 'so I gave them to her last night. She slept for three hours, the most she has had lately.' She looks desperate and, for the first time, touched by panic.

'It must be the morphine,' I say, trying to assuage her fears. She needs a full investigation, I chide myself. You don't need to be an oncologist to know that the combination of severe headaches and intractable vomiting raises the strong suspicion of secondary cancer in the brain. Having no idea how much of the disease Mrs Habib has on board, it is hard to predict, just from looking at her, how likely or unlikely she is to harbour cancer in the brain.

Not for the first time, I think longingly of what I could offer Mrs Habib if she had the good fortune not to be a refugee. I would admit her, treat her headache with powerful drugs, attach her to an intravenous drip to replenish her lost fluids, order urgent blood tests and a CT scan, and reassure the family that we would soon have an answer. To poor Mrs Habib, would this seem to be an overwhelming and unreal world of care?

The nurse sets about the herculean task of finding a lab that will run some basic tests free of cost. Most claim it is against policy or simply refuse. Then, with patient and daughter watching, I receive an astonishing phone call. It is a pharmacist on the line and he comes straight to the point.

'I am the pharmacist who sent you the Tamoxifen. My colleagues are warning me that I could be deregistered for giving Tamoxifen to a refugee.'

'Did we fail to pay you?' I ask to clear the confusion.

'No, no. I just shouldn't have done it. My job could be jeopardised.' He sounds chastened but goes on. 'I have to get it back, doctor.'

'I will make sure you get it back immediately.'

He sounds surprised, but relieved at the lack of resistance that he must have expected. I am far too dismayed to argue with him.

'And can I just say one more thing, doctor? You sound young. You might want to consider how far you want to go helping these people.'

Appalled and incredulous, I fling the unused Tamoxifen that the mortified daughter hands me back into a carton, where it lands amidst the near-expired bunch of donated asthma inhalers that the pharmacist had added in.

'Thank God my mother doesn't understand English,' the daughter whispers. Anger, shame and remorse clash in my head.

'We will get some Tamoxifen,' I promise her. 'Don't worry.'

I return to the phone with a vengeance and through sheer perseverance track down a radiologist who agrees to sign off on a free CT scan of her brain. I am grateful that he does this without any accompanying fanfare and I tell him so. 'I was once an immigrant myself,' he says by way of explanation.

Mrs Habib's men, as I have taken to calling them, bundle her up and take her straight to the radiology offices. When she returns with a normal report I am both relieved and disappointed. I have needlessly exhausted a precious favour. The thought makes me feel petty.

Mrs Habib's vomiting persists. It takes another week for the nurse to organise for a pathology laboratory to undertake her blood tests. Once again, the common thread is the migrant background of the owner. The blood tests reveal her to be anaemic and mildly dehydrated, but I am relieved that there is nothing else that could spell a medical emergency.

In the months ahead, under the grateful watch of her daughter, the clinic dips into its meagre donated funds for a panoply of anti-nausea drugs, morphine and nutritional drinks as the family resigns itself to her troublesome symptoms as a reality of cancer. Her deterioration happens so quickly that I decide to stop buying Tamoxifen and use the money to keep her comfortable instead. But just as her nausea abates, the relentless advance of the cancer brings forth another challenge. She comes in with excruciating hip pain and an X-ray reveals her hip to be eroded by cancer. She is in urgent need of radiotherapy.

I resign myself to yet another round of phone calls. I start with the doctors I know, confident that they will not demur in these disastrous circumstances. I am wrong. Everyone agrees that she needs radiotherapy but produces a reason why it cannot be done at their establishment. I am stunned out of my naivety. Finally, after two days of trying, I strike luck. One radiation oncologist agrees to treat Mrs Habib, but not before scoffing, 'Don't you think it's a little ironic that your large and famous hospital can't come to your rescue?'

I remain quiet, content to celebrate a minor feat rather than rue a worn irony. As we give Mrs Habib enough morphine to negotiate the journey to the radiation therapist in the back of a cramped car, it seems inappropriate to remark just how lucky she is.

'This clinic has been our saviour,' the daughter says. 'I can't imagine how stuck we would have been without you people.'

Mrs Habib has her radiotherapy with good effect although afterwards she becomes even more dependent on her family. Confined to a room in the small upstairs apartment the family shares, she is no longer able to attend my appointments, so I see only her daughter, who comes each week with a faithfully written diary about every single dose of morphine her mother has needed.

'I just feel like I need to show you this,' she says. I am struck by her integrity.

We display an air of nonchalance and I keep writing scripts for Mrs Habib's drugs to be dispensed by the local pharmacy, but the nurse and I privately wonder how much longer we can continue.

'One more cancer patient like her and that will be the end of us,' she declares morosely, staring into the nearly empty rickety drug cupboard. I know the clinic is financially strapped.

Then one week, the daughter fails to come. There can only be one reason.

'My mum passed away,' she says when she contacts me some time later. My heart sinks. I knew it was anticipated but the announcement of Mrs Habib's death underscores my failure to fulfil her needs.

'I am so sorry.'

'My family feels that the two of you were a godsend to my mother. What would we have done without you?' Never has such effusive praise felt so undeserved.

It is only after Mrs Habib's death that the pace of my afternoons at the clinic returns to normal. I go back to treating common infections, cuts and bruises, checking blood pressures and managing diabetes, all less onerous tasks than tackling cancer. It is only after her day-to-day problems have seeped out of my consciousness that the acrimonious discussion with my oncologist boss about doing research creeps back in. I am forced to acknowledge that here, in this refugee clinic, the things I *do* are actually quite few. The rest of the time I listen. I observe a lawyer's painful and humiliating transformation into an uncertain refugee, a teacher's slow internal death as she remembers terrifying events from her past and a young man's soured dreams. Neither an infant dehydrated from diarrhoea nor a pregnant refugee with syphilis will prove the subject of even an intriguing case report, let alone serious research. The renewal of blood pressure drugs or the treatment of dandruff is barely exalted fare, I think wryly, certainly nothing that a journal as hallowed as the *New England Journal of Medicine* would be interested in.

A knock on my door truncates my self-pity. A little boy has badly hurt his ankle in a fall, I am told. Will I wait to see him? Dusk has fallen and the area is unsafe. The obviously drug-crazed people outside look menacing. I hesitate for a second, enough for the nurse to offer, 'I will stay with you. She is coming from a long way. Do you have to go back to work after this?'

'No, I don't need to be back till the morning. I can stay.'

As I wait, the still-fresh memory of an unanticipated and bitter exchange that occurred only a few days ago comes into focus. This is my first year of being a trainee oncologist. So far, I have spent ten years in medical training, first as a student, and then as a doctor in the public hospital system. The next three years will take me through specialist training, at the end of which I will be a qualified oncologist. This is the minimum training one requires to be a specialist physician. It takes even longer to qualify as a surgeon. The long years of learning, the rigorous qualifying exams and the many personal sacrifices along the way mean that it requires resilience and a real belief in one's goals to keep going.

The actual transition to becoming a trainee oncologist has occurred in one sleep. One day I am a junior registrar reliant on a supervising consultant; the next day I am the first port for fielding calls about cancer patients, widely acknowledged to be some of the sickest and neediest. The phone calls come from the emergency department, where someone has landed with severe pneumonia and is near death. Should this man be resuscitated or allowed to die comfortably? In a remote feeder town, a patient has presented to the only doctor, unable to walk. He suspects her breast cancer has caused spinal cord compression – a true medical emergency. If she is not treated urgently, she will be paralysed. Could I arrange her immediate transfer, possibly by air ambulance?

'In this tiny town, I don't see much of this stuff,' the avuncular-sounding doctor explains somewhat apologetically as I walk him through the basics of treating his patient. 'In fact,' he says, 'unlike you, I have never seen a cord compression in my forty years of being a country doctor.' I have to suppress a laugh to uphold his misplaced faith in my expertise.

The first few weeks and months of advanced training can be a particularly important time, as expectations intersect with reality. I quickly discover what I had already guessed – that there are no easy patients and no simple deliberations in oncology. But I am relieved that, despite being thrown headlong into the daily care of these complex patients, the answers to whose questions I have yet to learn, I enjoy the essential dialogue. My favourite times are spent in the clinic, talking and listening to patients, discussing treatment options and managing the complications of therapy. Very early on, I recognise the privilege of being asked to be involved in some of the most momentous decisions in the lives of patients – decisions about starting and stopping treatment, making the final will, reconciling with an errant child. Many of my exchanges are uplifting and inspiring, despite being far too short. Many more are knotty or downright arduous, but time and again, they all illustrate the reason I chose to become a doctor and an oncologist – to witness the human condition up close, at its most vulnerable, and to be of practical help. I am relieved because though one's preferences in medicine can, over time, be calibrated, not so the fundamental passion for the profession.

Some months into my job, I survey the list of research projects I could start now and continue through the next few years. It is not a strict requirement at this stage of my training, but strongly recommended to improve the chances of securing a better job in the future. In addition to the standard specialist qualification, research credentials have become increasingly important in reaching the higher echelons of academic institutions that pride themselves on practising cutting-edge medicine. There are patient charts that need to be reviewed to tease out reasons why chemotherapy fails in certain patients, or to reveal ways to combat nausea better; retrospective data that need excavating from the bowels of the medical records office in order to track whether patients are living longer since the advent of newer treatments, and budding ideas for diagnosing cancer in its early phases. Nothing catches my attention. I know from watching my father's career as a theoretical physicist that research ideas need nurturing with genuine interest, tremendous patience and, often, a maniacal belief in their worth. I tell myself that I cannot do an honest job of summoning any of these qualities to the list before me and I feel doomed.

'So what do you think?'

My fresh copy of the list of research topics is still warm from the printer as I stand before my boss. He is an eminent man with a most impressive résumé. He seems genuinely knowledgeable and gets around difficult situations by calling on a ready recipe of solutions. He is able to recite from memory an infinite number of chemotherapy regimens and when I can't find them in the protocol book that I carry everywhere, he can grandly and truthfully claim that he has used the drugs with great satisfaction on his patients in a career spanning the best part of several decades. On such occasions, when my lack of experience is highlighted, I regard his with a mixture of veneration and fear. Is such acumen merely a result of the passage of enough time, or a reflection of intrinsic talent, bequeathed to the chosen?

I force my attention back to the piece of paper in my hands as I stand before his desk.

'Do you know what you are interested in?'

'Patients?' I ask tentatively, knowing that's not the right answer.

'No, no. I mean, what else? Have you found something else?'

Not yet, I guiltily admit. I am still finding my feet.

'I see.'

Warming up, I am quick to reassure him that I am relishing my job in oncology. 'It is just that I am interested in so many aspects of medicine.' A chance look behind him at the customised shelves brimming with texts, journals and publications evokes a surge of inadequacy in me, propelling me to say, 'I am not sure I want to go into research.' The release within me feels like a very loud roar. I wonder if he can hear it too.

Finely disseminated disapproval stares back at me. Opportunities abound in large institutions and it is up to me to grasp them. Surely, he finally says, a person seemingly motivated like me would know that the true measure of a physician comes from academic accomplishment. To gain even a modicum of standing within the medical profession, I must publish. An achievable goal should be writing a paper or two for every year of training, and publishing them in any journal, no matter how lowly ranked. The idea ought to be to set up a trail, perhaps culminating one day in a paper for the distinguished *New England Journal of Medicine*.

'In this day of competitive medicine, publishing is the only way ahead,' he remarks sagely, apparently without any reserve about the fundamental logic of his advice.

My eyes widen. The feeling of failure is never far from the minds of doctors. One's achievement is never enough, there being no lack of opportunity to cast a wry glance at what could have been. One's own achievement appears especially dubious when measured against the accomplishments of the profession, whose collective thirst for knowledge and advancement is legendary. I feel cornered but also slightly irritated at the meekness with which I must accept the implied criticism that choosing not to forge an early research career will consign me to the dustbin of medicine. Do I heed the disconcerting voice of wisdom or simply find the conviction to walk away? I am twenty-nine years old. For the first time in my life, I really don't know where to go.

'Sometimes you just need to find the will to start.'

He is right.

'In fact, I *am* working on a project.'

'Good! What is it?'

'I volunteer at a local refugee centre where I see patients who are denied access to medical care.' Interpreting his silence as approval, I warm to the topic. 'It is hard to believe some of the cases I see. It is certainly a world away from here . . .'

The kaleidoscope of expressions on his face travels quickly from bemusement to puzzlement to disdain. His reaction is swift, as if to quickly disavow me of a dangerous tendency. Such a pursuit is hardly academic, unlikely to win peer support or accolades. Moreover, it is simply irrelevant to my training as a cancer specialist. What is the point, he asks, of coming to a fine institution and then not advancing one's career in the tradition of eminent doctors?

I know in this instant that I have lost all credibility in the eyes of the man who only a few months ago hand-picked me from a field of distinctly qualified applicants. I have let him down, not so much by reprehensible conduct as flawed intent, perhaps made less forgiveable by its premeditated nature. But as I stand before him, made vulnerable by my own confession, I feel let down too. I thought he had the age and the cumulative experience to breathe life into my efforts, not douse them with discouragement, but it turns out that the high walls of the hospital have narrowed his field of vision too. His definition of a good physician is one who excels in a narrow area. I have met these so called sub-specialists too, like the orthopaedic surgeon who only operates on ankles or the cardiologist who specialises in fitting pacemakers. They have an important place in medicine, but surely, I think, we are a broad enough church to have room for the rest.

My mind floats back to the surgeon in my small Indian hometown, with whom I spent my elective as a medical student. If he chose simply to ply his trade narrowly, he would not help even a fraction of the people who flock to his clinic every day. But by being a family practitioner – part physician and part counsellor – he makes a disproportionate difference to the lives of his patients. Perhaps this is not how that septuagenarian imagined his life would unfold when he trained under some of England's finest specialists, but does his varied and sometimes pedestrian work somehow dilute his value as a doctor? And if so, in whose eyes? Certainly not for those who travel to see him and find solace in his attentive care.

And not in the eyes of the impoverished parents who intone their blessings upon him for saving their child from the clutches of diarrhoea or a skin infection turned gangrenous.

With nothing left to lose, I continue. 'The refugees are often sicker than hospitalised patients and completely disenfranchised. I want to write about my work with them.'

He emphatically tells me to leave this work to others and to concentrate instead on writing a scientific paper or starting a project. Kindness has never been a prerequisite for academic greatness, I am advised. Prestigious institutions will ask about the papers I never wrote, the research I never undertook, and I will soon find myself at a dead end.

'Think about it.' The statement sounds more warning than advice.

Piqued by the unanticipated reception, I feel akin to an errant child facing the unmasked irritation of quietly suffering parents. The chilly air blasts my face. The encounter is over. Pronounced unemployable by future institutions, frowned upon by the present, I leave the room full of questions. Was that the voice of wisdom trying to pull me back into the security of academic medicine before it is too late? Will my list of publications remain a distant dream, dwarfed by every one of my achieving peers who did as told? Am I destined to be an underachiever if I hit thirty without a scientific paper to my name? My passionate defences slowly evaporate, replaced by a forlorn feeling. I am jolted by the grim sentence, which threatens to be carried out in only a matter of time.

'Tell them you will enrol in a PhD in a couple of years,' a friend advises. 'You don't have to love everything you do and it gets them off your back.'

'It just doesn't seem right,' I protest.

'You can't always be idealistic,' she argues.

Straying from the norm is lonely at the best of times, especially when one is young and unsupported by the strength of one's own conviction. Should I be different? Why do I need to be different? Is it easier to join the pilgrimage demanded of me, although I know that only some travellers achieve the desired outcome while others are left to aspire to wear the mantle of greatness? And crucially, can there be a different aim to being a doctor and, if so, do institutions that pride themselves on their academic rigor eschew this aim for a reason? What defines a good doctor? One whose qualifications spill over the line or one whose patients are the most satisfied? And moreover, who defines a good doctor? In my heart of hearts, I have never been more convinced that I am doing the right thing, but even the stoutest resolve can unexpectedly stumble on doubt. I can't google the answer to my own questions.

The clinic nurse pops her head in, interrupting my extended reverie. 'Sorry, she is taking longer than I thought. It is just that if her son has fractured something he will need all your help to get him into a hospital.'

'Don't worry, I am going nowhere.'

And as I wait, I realise that medical research is not about to lose its vigour for my lack of direct participation, but what would the refugee centre do if its volunteers pulled out to engage in more 'academically worthy' work? There is nothing pedestrian about the day-to-day care of patients, refugees or otherwise. This is the kind of routine care that my family and I did not have when I was a child growing up in India. When my mother fell sick, it wasn't the doctors' lack of knowledge but a lapse in its application somewhere that debilitated and nearly killed her. Since no firm diagnosis was ever reached, there was no specific treatment either. She survived due to luck and her youth. But I saw that what helped her most was the extraordinary diligence of a man known as the 'compounder', a man with no formal qualifications who acquired his name from being part doctor, part pharmacist, part folk-healer; a man who had 'compounded' the skills he had picked up from observing the professionals. The compounder came every day, felt her pulse, touched her skin, talked to her and gave her hope. He administered the injections she needed but, mostly, he showed a true and touching interest in her welfare. When she recovered from the mysterious condition that had rendered her bed-bound for months, thought to be an adverse drug reaction, the compounder's joy rivalled my family's. What ordinary people want is a doctor who will listen to their problems and treat them with humanity and decency. These skills are honed not in the laboratory but by sitting with patients.

The little boy arrives with his mother. He is six years old and frightened. The nurse bribes him with a crayon to let me examine his ankle. I am satisfied that it is not broken. The nurse congratulates his mother for having applied ice to the bruise.

'I will drive you home, it's on my way,' the nurse offers. The mother nods gratefully. There is relief written over all our faces.

As we walk out into the night, I tell myself then that maybe I will not pen my first scientific paper for years to come. Who knows, I may never get around to writing one! And my boss is probably right that there will be institutions that will not welcome me past their threshold. But if I replace all the scientific papers with scribbled notes about refugees, dispossessed and at the mercy of volunteers, I doubt that it will be a wasted career. And if I never earn the title of professor, but practise my profession with kindness and humility, I will be content in the knowledge that I am not losing anything nearly as precious as every one of my patients whose history lies before me on sheets of recycled paper.

4

◇

You are the doctor

He could be a doting grandfather, relishing an afternoon in the lush green of the park, or a devoted husband or concerned father. Yet today he is only my patient, in a windowless consulting room, far from capable of relishing anything. He usually addresses me as 'doctor' but sometimes he trips up and calls me 'darling'. He does this so naturally that I have never had the heart to object.

He is nearly eighty years old and has never been sick until developing liver metastases six months ago. Since the incidental diagnosis, made when he faithfully went to his doctor for a flu shot, he has undergone exhaustive investigations to locate the primary cancer, subjected his mind to weeks of waiting and last-minute consultations, his body to all manner of uncomfortable tests. In the meantime he has developed extensive deep vein thrombosis, an ominous sign of the resolutely obscure yet aggressive cancer. But remarkably, he has continued to feel well, dampening my initial urgency to treat him. He knows that in this situation, any chemotherapy is designed to palliate not cure. 'I feel okay so what is the point in not feeling so okay?' encapsulates the Eastern European stoicism that I will come to identify as his trademark. But my colleagues and I keep ordering scans and documenting progressive disease, ultimately succeeding in contaminating his calm with our concern. So one day, after we have repeatedly posed the same question – 'Do you feel like having treatment? We could treat you if you wanted,' – he ventures, 'I suppose I could try some chemotherapy, see if it does me any good.'

My first reaction to this response is disappointment. 'I was just doing my job,' I want to extract myself from the process by saying. 'You don't have to listen to everything I say.' But to patients who hang on the doctor's every facial expression, let alone the spoken word, this would seem incomprehensible. In fact, I can almost hear him shake his head in confusion. 'Lady, why would you talk to me about chemotherapy if you don't want me to have it?'

Because I am a newly minted oncologist and I feel that in order to be a successful physician, my conversations must be accompanied by a demonstration of my knowledge about the primary tool of my trade, chemotherapy. This has been my medical upbringing. During my training, hardly anyone, even those with advanced disease and a poor constitution, was flatly refused chemotherapy. Many patients, obviously poor candidates for tolerating its toxic rigours, were prescribed treatment, perhaps with smaller doses or at increased intervals. We felt uncertain about some of our decisions, expressing little hope of benefit, warning our colleagues to look out for early signs of harm, but we signed off on the chemotherapy. I talked to many of these patients and witnessed many more consultations. I saw that it took far less time to dictate the list of anticipated side effects from chemotherapy than to enter into a discussion about one's broader goals in life and why the statistician's definition of a significant prolongation of survival seldom translated into individual patient gratification. It was also less emotionally taxing to hold out hope by the slenderest of threads by offering a whiff of chemotherapy than to confront one's impotence as a doctor.

The reasons for offering treatment that was most likely going to prove futile were always the same. It was the principle of autonomy – the patient got to be the final arbiter. Anything less was paternalism, the curse of ancient medicine, when the doctor sat in judgement, and the doctor's word was final. And who were doctors to deny a patient the small, barely existent chance of a particular treatment working, even if they had never before beheld such a miracle? Then there were the angry relatives, banging on the door for something, anything, to be done. Something needed to be done to pacify them too. And finally, the patient was only trying chemotherapy, with complete freedom to stop it at any stage if the side effects mounted.

The principles may have sounded okay, but in real life what I saw was patients taking risks out of desperation, tolerating terrible side effects out of obligation, continuing treatment out of an inability to decide. The same relatives who had been pounding the door returned woebegone to say they never understood that chemotherapy had the greatest chance of not working; the same patient who had expressed a desire to try 'something, anything', now wished we had explicitly told him it was a bad idea.

'If I really understood what a small response rate meant, I would have never come back.'

But this was modern medicine at its best, its most giving. Well-trained doctors were meant to be dispassionate dispensers of options and sellers of hope. Not for them to shake their head and say there was nothing else in their armoury of drugs, for that would be confessing to ignorance or, worse, failure.

The consultations I most enjoyed watching and being part of were the difficult medical and ethical ones, which required more finesse than knowledge; the ones where the oncologist virtually needed to save a patient from his own false expectations. I could see that with patience and a strong concern for overall patient welfare, doctors could manoeuvre patients through genuinely fraught decisions about their health, talk them into therapy when needed, but also out of treatment when appropriate.

'Patients are not fools,' an oncologist once explained to me after a long discussion ending in the decision to opt for palliative care. The patient had presented us with a pile of internet printouts about his advanced cancer, with statistics that sounded promising only until his individual poor prognosis was made clear. 'But patients are not doctors either. You and I are, and sometimes we *do* know best.' At the time, I marvelled to myself that only his grey hair gave him the licence to make such a grand, paternalistic claim, but he was actually providing me with one of the more useful lessons in the art of being a doctor.

'So you are sure about having chemotherapy?' I ask my patient now.

'After all the talk, let's give it a go.'

He is unconvinced. So am I. But it gives us both something to do.

Predictably, the chemotherapy achieves exactly what I dreaded – multiple side effects without any benefit. He vomits regularly, he loses the power of taste, his appetite fades and he spends more and more time in bed. When he becomes anaemic, we transfuse him with blood, but the warm red of the blood does not reproduce itself in the pale hollow of his cheeks. He throws up the anti-nausea drugs in the bucket he carries with him wherever he goes. The next scan is his worst ever. It is almost as if the disease, offended by the assault, has decided to raise its head even more ferociously, showing what it can really do.

Despite the setbacks during the few cycles of chemotherapy, he remains philosophical, even warm and affable towards the staff. His wife always accompanies him, never failing to impress me with the way she juggles multiple appointments, home visits by nurses, the administration of his pills, regular blood tests and countless phone calls. About the same age as him, their physical appearances have changed considerably since he began to lose weight and condition. She is still a healthy and able seventy, although I wonder what mental toll this ordeal must be exacting on her. But if she finds this stressful, she is not going to confess to it now. When he rambles during his appointments with me, as he is increasingly prone to do, her eyes seek mine as if to apologise, yet she unfailingly respects his need to talk. She never interrupts him, even when I wish she would. In time, I grow to admire this very ability she possesses to be tolerant – we could all do with more of the skill.

Today they have come in for an unscheduled appointment, concerned about his plummeting state. Alarmingly, he arrives on a stretcher. He has never let us arrange transport, claiming it is for really sick patients and those who have no help. 'I have still got the wife, don't you worry!' he would say, good-naturedly dismissing my concerns as he patted his wife's hand.

His abdominal pain is worse and he has not eaten in days. He looks pale, gaunt and spent. She is exhausted, not having slept for several nights because he has started to wander in confusion. His weakness places him at risk of falls. I can see from her face that she does not expect to have him around for long.

Annoyed at myself, I say, 'I don't think the chemotherapy is working; in fact, it seems to be making you worse.' Then I bite my tongue, thinking I ought to have asked him his opinion first. His wife throws me an acquiescing glance while he simply shrugs his shoulders. I brace myself for reasoning and counter-reasoning, pleas, anger, but there is only silence followed by that familiar conciliatory tone: 'You are the doctor.' Immediately I doubt my judgement. Is he just having a bad day or week? Given time, will chemotherapy triumph over his deadly symptoms? Have I just traded his hope for presumed quality of life? I wish he would challenge my assertion, telling me I may be the doctor but I don't know everything. That since I talked him into having chemotherapy in the first place, he expects me to reverse his symptoms and return him to his old health. I won't be able to deliver on his demand but at least it will provide me with a chance to express my regret. But he has sunk back into his cold, narrow stretcher, his eyes shut, his hand closing over his bulging, painful liver.

Under the transparent bed sheet his grossly swollen, clotted leg appears continuous with his engorged abdomen. It is hard to believe the leg has been able to bear any of his weight lately, or that its constant pain has responded more than marginally to pain-killers. Since he looks to be asleep, I start talking with his wife about the logistics of palliative care. But he soon wakes, and at the mention of diabetes exclaims, 'Diabetes! Oh, let me tell you about the diabetes. I thought I had avoided the curse but let me tell you what it's done to me.'

He proceeds to lead me through the various drugs he has tried to offset the rise in his blood sugars caused by the steroids prescribed for his nausea. The readings have swung wildly, the highs making him feel manic, the lows plunging his vision into darkness.

'Where is the logbook, darling?' he asks his wife. 'The doctor needs to see it.'

'Don't worry,' she soothes. 'I think she gets the idea.'

'Oh, I don't think so. Does she know the reading was thirty today?'

'It was three,' she corrects him wearily. 'Because you haven't eaten since yesterday.'

'Oh. Well, three then. It's still bad.'

The recollection of this and other aspects of his daily routine is rendered difficult by his unreliable memory and staccato speech. I glance at my watch, reminded of the waiting room filling up with patients, but he shows no sign of stopping.

'The insulin pen. What do we do about getting another one?'

'You don't need one,' I respond. 'Your sugars are running low.'

'Hmm . . . but what if they go high again?'

I am surprised by his lucidity, especially for one who looked so seriously ill that I had thought him incapable of any useful conversation. But part of me is also impatient, because this involved discussion about insulin seems pointless in the larger scheme of things. Aware that this is almost certainly our last meeting, I feel caught between serving a dying patient and helping the living. The longer I spend with him the greater the chance that someone waits outside with unmanaged pain, troublesome nausea or unresolved apprehension. Fighting an emerging hint of resentment at being trapped, I excuse myself to fetch some letterhead.

'I need to write to your nurses.'

When I re-enter the room he recommences with gusto. 'You know, my cousin has diabetes. I just found out. You think the cancer made my diabetes appear? Or does diabetes give you cancer?'

'Remember we looked it up on the internet? Diabetes doesn't cause cancer,' his wife soothes, doing her best to engage him.

I avert my head, writing a detailed note to the palliative care team about his imminent decline. His wife sits patiently between us. How many times has she heard him go off on a tangent? How does she make conversation so well?

Absorbed in writing and becoming increasingly disinterested,

I answer only in monosyllables but he does not seem to care. Then, as my pen comes to a halt, so does his reminiscing. He says with a start, 'I am sorry! I just kept going and took up all your time. How long have I been here? I don't feel so well. Can I have some morphine?'

'That's okay,' I reassure him, struggling to appear gracious in front of his wife, witness to my fidgeting for the past half-hour. She reaches into her bag for the bottle of morphine. His eyelids flutter to a close in anticipation of a temporary reprieve from pain.

'Sometimes he does this.' His wife says this softly but contritely. It is difficult to miss the ever-deepening bags under her eyes; they scream of sleeplessness. 'You just have to let him talk himself out. Thank you.'

Guiltily I seek to redeem myself by walking to his side. 'Is there anything else you would like me to know about your diabetes, or any other worries?'

He takes my hand, which rests on the side of his bed. He makes an effort to arouse himself from sleep and says weakly but determinedly, 'Just that I appreciate your care and patience with me. You have been honest and I like that.'

I am left without words. I wonder if he is being sarcastic but he sounds sincere. His wife nods at me. 'He really means that.'

He closes his eyes and breathes deeply. I can't help noticing that his hand is still embracing his abdomen, as if to talk it into relaxing, not hurting so much.

I fold the letter to the home-care nurses and place it in an envelope.

'How are you doing?' I ask his wife. 'This must be hard.'

'You do what you have to do. It's part of being married.'

She says this simply, but there is nothing simple about her courage.

'Do you think you can do this at home?' I ask.

'It's what he wants and I have never thought otherwise.'

'You know there is hospice too, if you need it.'

'I would . . .'

Suddenly and unbelievably, he is wide awake and in full possession of his senses again as he directs his wife to take him home. 'Let's go, darling. We need to have lunch.'

'Yes, yes. The doctor was just finishing up.'

I wonder whether he had been watching us through half-closed eyes, listening in and interrupting when the mention of hospice must have sounded like I was threatening not to return him home. And it dawns on me that his launching into seemingly unrelated topics like his diabetes may have been his way of wrapping up his life, his clinic visits; of saying goodbye.

Aware of not wanting to create unnecessary fear, I tell him that I will call transport immediately. I tell him that it has been nice having him around today, and I wish him well. Unlike all the other times, he doesn't ask when he should make the next appointment and I don't suggest it. I want to say that I will miss his cheery smile and wave from the waiting room; instead, afraid to summon his demise, I ask his wife to call me if she needs me. My regret at having subjected him to futile chemotherapy stays on my lips.

'Darling, you have done all you could.' He smiles at me before closing his eyes again.

As the porter pushes out the stretcher, I reflect on the fact that of the many conversations we have had, this was the one that meant the most to him and the one that I did the least justice to. Our chats about what investigations to perform next used to be detailed and informative, but so disappointing in their yield. The discussions about chemotherapy were equally animated yet the treatment achieved little. And today, when he is near the end of his life, our conversation barely deserved to be called that. It was a monologue – his desire to call it a day doing battle with my unwillingness to facilitate it.

The next week, I receive a call from his wife. Her voice bears the heaviness of unmitigated sorrow. 'I called to tell you that he passed away. All our children came home in time. He said after his last clinic visit that he just knew he wasn't going back. And he said he would miss you in a way and to say thank you.'

Moved, I offer my condolences to her and extend an invitation to answer the family's questions if any emerge. I tell her how much I enjoyed looking after her husband and how I miss his face in the waiting room. As I speak I am stunned by the hollowness of my sincerity. I wish that instead of writing a letter to somebody else to assume his care, I had sat back and indulged his story about errant blood sugars and whatever else his heart desired. I think ruefully that this could have been our most gratifying interaction if only I had given it a chance. But we had remained worlds apart and now it is too late.

She hangs up in tears and I walk out to call the next patient. As I watch a frail and emaciated woman helped to her feet by her husband who is in equally poor condition, I know that there will be a next time to do things better.

5

◇

No harm in trying

The last patient in clinic does not show up. The secretary stands ready, brandishing a red stamp that screams FTA – failed to attend. I suppress a sigh of relief at finishing my work a little earlier than anticipated. It has been a busy morning and the occasional no-show provides a welcome respite. I glance at the list; noting Steven's name at the end, I don't pay it more attention. Absent patients can be a source of concern as well as extra work. At the end of each clinic, the secretary neatly lays out the files of those who failed to keep their appointment. Her job finishes there; she is unaware of the gravity of a patient's situation or the implications of a missed visit. So it falls to a doctor to review each file and decide how soon the patient must be recalled. Some clinics, such as the one which sees patients with advanced lung cancer, are routinely overbooked under the assumption that a handful of patients will die before their next review. The practice underscores the terrible scourge of lung cancer. However, when patients fail to show up to an early breast cancer clinic, it is equally likely that they omitted to reschedule an appointment or have gone away on vacation and forgotten their appointment. This is a rough but practical measure of the wellness of a patient and hence the seriousness with which to treat a particular non-attendance.

Steven has cancer of the pancreas. If it was another patient in his place, I may have made a phone call or asked the secretary to send out an urgent reminder, but Steven is one of my most reliable patients. I would not be surprised if he had called to change his appointment and the message didn't get through. Making nothing more of the matter, I move on to the pile of paperwork, which incidentally includes completing some more of Steven's insurance-claim forms, which I have finally convinced him to obtain.

Just then, the secretary pokes her head in. 'I just wanted to let you know that Steven died.'

'What? Are you sure?'

My heart immediately fills with dismay as I remember Steven, last seated before me only a few weeks ago. We spoke at length about his painkillers as we struggled to achieve an acceptable degree of comfort for him. He had winced and smiled alternatively throughout the consultation, believing that his youth gave him reason to be stoic but finding that his disease just kept getting the edge.

'I wouldn't feel so bad if you could just do something about the pain,' he would say again and again, before valiantly adding, 'But I guess you are, and that's the best you can do. Never mind.' Although he meant no criticism, his words always served to accentuate my failure to control his pain effectively.

'Yes,' the secretary answers, 'I found out from palliative care.'

'Thank you for letting me know.'

'I really liked him. What a shame.' She wipes away the tears from her eyes.

Death features ubiquitously in an oncology practice. From time to time, when I am signing a death certificate, I reflect on the fact that most other people in their thirties have often experienced only the death of their grandparents. Even among doctors, other specialists lose a patient infrequently compared to the oncologist or palliative-care physician. In only my first year of being an oncology trainee, I watched the deaths of more people than I did over the preceding decade. By the time I qualified, I too had learnt to react to the news of the death of a patient with characteristic nonchalance, wary of tapping into the true extent of my emotion in public.

'Oh, that's sad,' I might mutter sometimes if the secretary or a nurse lingers in the room, beginning to leaf distractedly through whatever notes are lying before me. I have discovered this is a good way to discourage further conversation about the deceased. An attuned secretary or nurse will often command a better grasp than the doctor of the more human attributes of the patient – who brought her in to her consultations, how many times he had to wait more than an hour, when she first realised that chemotherapy was not working. It is hard to be reminded of this gulf between the patient and doctor.

Other times, especially in conversation with another oncol-ogist, one of us might say, 'He had a terrible disease to begin with,' as if this bleak pronouncement assuages the fatal outcome or even justifies the length of time the patient actually survived. But when one works with desperately ill patients every day, it becomes necessary to reconcile quickly with their loss and look ahead to helping the next person.

I look up to find the secretary holding Steven's file.

'I thought you might need this.' She has worked here long enough to know that I would like a phone number from his file.

Steven was different from the outset. For a start, at thirty-seven, he seemed too young to develop an incurable cancer. While I celebrated impending parenthood, he was losing weight and developing worsening abdominal pain. When his symptoms first appeared, he attributed them to erratic eating because his wife had started classes at the local music school, leaving him to make his own dinner on many nights. But once she noticed his weight loss, his explanation did not seem sound and she urged him to see his doctor. Unlike some instances where it can take weeks for a diagnosis to be made, Steven's doctor faxed me a letter the same afternoon. It said, 'Please see this young man presenting with an enlarged, painful liver and weight loss. Tests confirm cancer of the pancreas with liver secondaries.'

Steven was placed in the urgent slot the very next morning. He came alone. The history was brief, in keeping with that of a previously healthy young man. No, he did not have any notable medical conditions. He did not smoke, use drugs or alcohol. His parents were in their early seventies and currently on a walking tour overseas, making full use of their exemplary fitness. He had never heard of cancer in even a distant relative. He had been married to Lisa, several years younger than him, for five years; she now felt ready to start a family. He had led an interesting life so far. A well-regarded swimmer, he used to be a surf club lifesaver before changing occupations completely to become a miner. He had nurtured a childhood fascination with mines and found work in a coal mine an hour out of town. There, he met two long-lost school mates. The three men were responsible for maintaining electrical equipment in the mine. He felt as if he couldn't ask for a better deal than working with two friends in a job of his choosing.

I remember telling him the diagnosis as if it were yesterday. Although his family doctor has warned him, he is taken aback to hear it confirmed by me. He is even more stunned to hear that his disease is incurable.

'Shit,' he swears, before covering his mouth. 'I am sorry, doc.' Sweat breaks out on his temples.

I regard him in silence. Metastatic pancreatic cancer is a terrible disease, the prognosis for which has remained resolutely dismal over the years. With this enormous burden, I know that he is going to enter trouble rapidly.

At first, surprisingly, he is ambivalent about having chemotherapy. I think that perhaps I have not explained clearly enough, or he has failed to understand the ominous implications of his disease, but after the second consultation, he concludes that chemotherapy is his only hope of earning even a short reprieve.

'I guess there's no harm in trying,' he says, with the understated practicality that I will soon come to identify with him.

There is in fact the potential for plenty of harm from therapy but the alternative is no more acceptable, so we go ahead. Steven tolerates the first few weeks of chemotherapy reasonably well but soon the side effects begin to mount. He is ravaged by nausea and vomiting and then frequent bouts of pain in his abdomen. At each consultation, he states these facts plainly, without apparent emotion or embellishment. I sometimes think that he recites his symptoms with the same degree of interest as one would a familiar bus timetable.

'That doesn't sound good,' I prompt, trying to gauge how much his symptoms bother him.

'They are okay. It's just the first few days and then I'm back to work.'

'If you say so.'

A cancer clinic is usually so packed with malcontent patients with upsetting concerns that one begins to unconsciously appreciate the occasional upbeat exchange. Although it does not mitigate one's awareness of the suffering the majority of patients experience during cancer treatment, the occasional patient who bullishly asserts his well-being can be a welcome antidote. I could push Steven harder about his symptoms but I don't want to. It seems so much nicer and easier to believe that he is doing as well as he states.

A further few weeks into treatment, Steven's symptoms worsen. He keeps his appointments faithfully but I can tell that he is beginning to struggle. I wonder what motivates him to continue in the face of such poor quality of life. Is he clinging to an overly optimistic expectation of benefit? Have I misled him somewhere along the way? Is he desperate to live long enough so that Lisa and he can have a child? He faces the treatment with such resolve that I cannot find the heart to broach these obvious questions. But with every passing week, I wonder what role I play by signing off on another round of treatment.

Somewhat uncharacteristically, Steven's pain never lessens. He describes it as 'stable bad' on most days and 'really awful' on others. The morphine I prescribe causes constipation; the constipation, headache; the headache, insomnia and fatigue. But he keeps battling on. One day he requests a medical certificate.

'Sure. How many months should I make it for?'

'Just today, thank you.'

'What do you mean?'

'I take Friday afternoon off work to see you before I go straight to treatment. I recover on the weekend and go back to work on Monday.'

I look at him incredulously.

'You mean you have been working throughout chemotherapy?'

'Oh yes. What else would I do with my time?'

Feel sorry for yourself? I want to suggest. Wonder why you have the misfortune to be facing such a disease?

'But, Steven, that wouldn't give you much time to recover. That's tough!' I finally say.

'I am okay.'

But now he has me worried. Is he in denial about his poor prognosis? Is there another problem I haven't tapped into?

'Do you need the money? Is that why you work?'

'No!' he laughs. 'Lisa and I are doing well. I don't have to work but I like to. And if I stopped, people would worry about me.'

Unable to picture him performing manual labour safely down a mine-shaft, I urge him to stop working.

'I love my job as much as you love yours,' he responds with a smile. 'And I am not going to get any better by being home,' he adds sanguinely.

Somehow he makes sense by instilling an uncommon practicality into his dealings with a terminal illness. There are many adjectives to describe him – courteous, friendly, undemanding, strong – but I also just like him. He breaks up my day with his smile and his understated manner of describing his symptoms. And although I struggle to come to terms with his illness, he seems at peace with his prognosis and doesn't force me to dig for meaning. He comes to be treated by me, but I am the one who is left feeling better.

At his next visit, he looks distinctly more tired and I order a CT scan, fearing the result but hoping I am proven wrong. On the morning of his review, his films go missing, resulting in a two-hour wait while the nurse hunts them down. He doesn't complain once or make a snide remark about our inefficiency. When I finally put the films up on the viewing screen, the evidence of his decline is heartbreakingly obvious. The lumps in his liver have grown larger, coalescing into masses that all but obliterate any normally function-ing tissue. Even Steven's unpractised eye can draw circles around the lumps.

'Yes, it does look worse.' I nod my head slowly in agreement with him. 'But sometimes the pictures don't really match up with how you feel,' I offer, trying to soften the blow.

Like every other time, I expect him to maintain that he has experienced nothing but the usual troubles with which he has to deal. Or, I prepare myself, there may finally be dismay or anger that even after following the prescribed therapy with a near-devout attitude, he is still not winning. But nothing has prepared me for his rejoinder. Regarding the telltale films one more time, he exhales deeply. 'I can finally stop chemotherapy then.'

This response takes me by surprise. Thus far he has provided no indication that the chemotherapy has been difficult for him. He has not only been uncomplaining but has strived to play down the severity of his obvious symptoms. And now, here he is, in an apparent rapid reconciliation with his cursed fate, as if he expected it all along but has simply been humouring me by undergoing treatment.

'I don't think this chemotherapy has done you any favours,' I reluctantly admit.

But he is just too young to die and although I have yet to see a good outcome from pancreatic cancer, I desperately want him to be the first.

'Steven, I am sorry. I am going to call around to see what else I can do.'

He shrugs his shoulders, his usually pleasant expression clouded by doubt.

People often accuse oncologists of being miserly when it comes to lending hope, but no one appreciates how difficult it can be sometimes to find that glimmer of hope to give to a patient. No one more than me wants to tell Steven that the progression of his cancer is a temporary setback. I want to say that there are other means to trick his disease; that even if I cannot banish the cancer, I can turn it into an annoying but bearable hanger-on. But in truth, his cancer is so vengeful that it would immediately spurn all such dreamy pronouncements. He knows this.

However, I convince him to seek a second opinion. The oncologist he sees has nothing to offer him but I feel as if my guilt at the failure of my treatment has been fractionally absolved. Despite another devastating iteration of his prognosis, he returns with his unflappable calm intact.

'They said my liver is too full of cancer for any experimental drugs to work. They said they will put me on the books if something comes up.'

I study his face keenly, wondering whether he really believes that anything will come up. Does he live in false hope and does this explain his nonchalance? Or is he in denial and in need of psychological assistance? A high proportion of cancer sufferers have undiagnosed depression at some stage of their illness. I wonder if I am holding on to a depressed patient. Should I let him take the cue and ask me more meaningful questions or should I be more forthcoming in spelling out his condition? But in blaming shortcomings, his and mine, for his apparent lack of comprehension about his disease, I succeed in completely underestimating Steven. I have failed to recognise that this simple young man, neither highly educated nor well-connected, possesses an uncommon ability to cope with misfortune. My narrow vision will become obvious only in hindsight.

Unable to offer Steven any more useful therapy, I promise to concentrate on his quality of life. He makes it clear that he wants to keep working for as long as possible. But there is never any mention of dying. Unlike some other patients who have wanted to know in excruciating detail how the human body succumbs, Steven either doesn't care or doesn't care to know. I try a slightly different approach.

'What about your wife? What does she want?'

'She says she just wants me to be happy.'

I can't help but feel curious about Lisa, who has never once attended a consultation or called me to find out more. What is Steven telling her? Do I owe her any explanations if she is on the trail of suddenly finding her husband dead one day? I freeze at the recollection of one patient's wife who took me to task so spectacularly for having kept her in the dark after her husband died without ever having told her of his condition.

'Steven, why doesn't your wife come with you?'

'No offence, doc, but this is a pretty grim place,' he replies, pointing to my room. 'I don't want her to start mourning before she has to.' I am touched by his concern for his wife's well-being at a time when he could certainly do with additional support.

'Do you talk to her about how you feel? Does she know what's going on?'

'Oh, she knows. But my worries? I try to leave them underground, doc. Best place, I would say.'

Remarkably, Steven continues to work for the next two months. He cuts down the frequency of his consultations to avoid taking days off. I keep escalating his morphine and try numerous other painkillers in the hope of striking something that works. His gait grows awkward as he hunches over in pain, one hand nursing his abdomen. He refuses to accept the offer of a wheelchair to and from his car, asserting that other people need it more. Some days he carries a plastic bag stuffed in his pocket so that any involuntary wave of nausea won't soil his clothes. But throughout his visits, he retains his friendly greeting and straightforward descriptions of his symptoms.

Sometimes, I want to reach beneath the surface questions about pain, bowels and fatigue to see how he is coping emotionally. But although I find this natural enough to ask my elderly patients, I feel inhibited asking Steven how he feels about his imminent death. What if he says he is scared? Could I tell him I would be too?

What if he says he has many unfulfilled dreams? Unlike the ninety-year-old grandmother, how could I console him that he has led a rich life? If he tells me he really wants a child, would I be able to hide my remorse at his missing out on one of life's greatest gifts, one that I have only just begun to discover for myself?

Never quite confident as to what is most appropriate, I squander many opportunities to treat the whole person, instead choosing the easy option to focus on the disease. I feel terrible.

'How is it going?' a colleague asks me one day, perhaps noticing my distraction as we head to a meeting.

I think about telling her. But I realise that in all this time, I have never heard anyone else discuss anything that even remotely resembles how I felt about Steven. At our round-table meetings, we discuss challenging patients, debate interesting ones, provide conference updates and ponder career planning. But to the frequent question, 'Is there anything else we need to talk about?' no one has ever volunteered, 'I don't know that you can do anything, but I feel terrible about a patient.'

Having only recently qualified at this point and extremely mindful of my position as a junior specialist, I naively assume that everyone else has come upon a way of dealing with the existential questions that plague my conscience.

'Busy day,' I respond, biting into my sandwich.

'I know what you mean,' she says, unwrapping hers.

Inevitably, the day arrives when Steven is forced to leave work. 'I keep falling asleep in the mine and my friends just let me rest till it's time to go home. I used up a whole bottle of morphine syrup this week. I can't go on like this.'

Although I have been pressing him for months to leave work, I now experience more than a twinge of sadness at hearing him agree, for this really marks the beginning of the end. Instead of a medical certificate for the day, I fill out his life insurance forms, hoping that he has some weeks left to enjoy the proceeds of a lifetime of work. In the section titled 'Life Expectancy', I tick the box marked 'less than one month'. Even as I keep my eyes firmly fixed on the application, I wonder whether to broach the issue of his imminent death, but I waver at the last minute. His observant eyes take in everything on the form but all he says is, 'Thank you'. I don't sleep that night. I doubt that he does either.

The next week, impossibly, his pain is even worse. For the first time he calls me from home. 'I can't move,' he groans. 'I've run out of morphine and I am in too much pain.'

'Do you want me to call you an ambulance? Come straight to hospital.'

'No, please don't make me do this. I have had enough of hospitals. Can you just post me another script?'

Apart from doing what he asks, I arrange for an anaesthetist to perform a nerve block, a procedure that destroys the local nerves that signal pain. But Easter is approaching and the first available appointment is several weeks away.

'I am sorry,' I remark to Steven, exasperated at my impotence. A welcome respite for doctors, prolonged public holidays are a curse for patients like him.

'You are doing all you can,' he offers graciously.

I hate the way he is forced to sit for hours in the waiting room, retaining no individuality despite possessing the strength and courage of several men. His courteous and polite conduct makes his suffering all the more unbearable. Seeing Steven dispirits me, but not seeing him fills me with apprehension. I pray that the anaesthetist will make good on his promise to fit him into the first cancellation.

During Steven's wait for a nerve block, I receive a call from his wife, telling me that he is driving himself to the emergency room with uncontrolled pain.

'Save the ambulances for heart attacks and critical things. I have had pain for months and months,' he told the nurse who begged him to wait at home.

Although I have lost count of my consultations with Steven, I have never met Lisa.

'Steven said if anything happened, to call you.' She sounds afraid, in a panic.

I feel awkward asking her any questions, unsure of the extent of her knowledge. 'I will catch up with him in emergency,' I assure her.

When he stumbles up to the triage nurse, his liver failure is obvious. The staff are incredulous that a man in his condition had the strength to drive himself. He is rushed into a bed and is in such severe pain that he asks to be sedated. For once, the emergency doctors do not run the usual gamut of tests but simply honour his request. Just then, a bed in the hospice becomes available and Steven is transferred to its quieter surrounds. By the time I finish with patients and make it to the emergency department, the ambulance that he had never wanted to ride in has left with him fast asleep in the back.

In the hospice, he drifts in and out of sedation, smiles at his wife, and goes back to sleep. The physician worries that his pain is still not controlled but Steven resolutely refuses to complain, saying only that everyone is trying their best.

'It's not long to go now,' he whispers to the doctor one evening. 'This has been hard on everybody.'

The veteran hospice physician tells me that Steven is one of the most heroic patients he has ever met.

'The poor man, was he comfortable in hospice?' the nurse wants to know.

The hospice being only a few minutes down the road, I had every intention of visiting Steven, but my courage never went further than making phone enquiries about him. I felt unable to confront Steven, whom I saw as a personal representation of my failure. Never having met Lisa, I didn't think I could handle our first face to face meeting at the bedside of her dying husband. I left a message with his nurse but I don't know that anyone ever heard the dejection in my voice or read the urgency hidden in the benign message, 'Your doctor called'. I wondered later whether he even got my message and whether he asked himself why, after week upon week of following him so closely, I didn't bother to see him in his final days. He was never the sort who would demand attention, content to leave such decisions in the hands of others. And it was not as if I had offered him anything other than shattered expectations, although I hoped that I had been kind.

'I don't know,' I say contritely. 'I didn't make it there.'

'I am sure they looked after him well. He was a good guy.'

Her words remind me that he was indeed a good guy. As I stare at Steven's file and my notes scribbled across dozens of pages, I wish now that I had told him how much I admired his courage, without the fear of embarrassing either of us. I wish that just as he routinely and graciously expressed confidence in my treatment decisions, I had stated my respect for his spirited conduct in the face of a terrifying disease. I know now that a touch of his hand as he lay dying would have carried as much meaning as the tiresome visits where we talked response rates and clinical trials.

It is too late now. Reflexively, I dial his home number. There is no answer. I call his wife's phone. It is silent. I hesitate to call his mobile phone, not knowing what I will do at the tone. When I do,

Steven's voice sounds – strong, amicable, from a time when his world was predictable and the challenges surmountable. Following his instructions, I leave a message after the beep. 'Steven, you were pretty amazing. Your courage through difficult times was extraordinary and I am going to miss seeing you.'

I hang up self-consciously. The superstitious part of me hopes that he hears now what I should have told him a long time ago.

6

◇

I just want to talk

Although I have delayed seeing him till last, it is still early morning when I tiptoe into his room in the hospice. Stopping by the bedside, I gaze at his placid expression, debating whether to wake him for a desultory conversation or allow him his much-needed rest. The pallor of his smooth-shaven face is tinged by a shade of yellow that grows deeper by the day. The thin bed sheet does little to obscure the gross swelling of his legs and scrotum, now weeping their contents onto the mattress. The urinary catheter has taken on a fluorescent hue, a contrast to the flaccid bag of dull saline that has dripped aimlessly away. Yet, despite the signs of discomfort, he breathes peacefully and I decide against waking him. As I pick up his chart, the hard folder clangs noisily against the cold metal of his bed and before I know it, he is awake and I am sorry.

'I didn't mean to wake you, Dr Harding,' I apologise.

'You are early,' he greets me weakly, letting his eyes adjust.

'How are you feeling today?'

'My leg has almost no pain. It's amazing,' he says, shifting cautiously but not really moving at all. His eyes divulge his pain.

'Can I get you something to make you a bit more comfortable?'
I ask solicitously.

'I am going to wait a bit. I am fed up with these pills.'

He was about to start teaching a new batch of medical students
when he developed a pain in his lower abdomen. Having just
returned from a holiday to Vietnam, he went to his family practitioner, suspecting hepatitis acquired from the street fare he
had happily indulged in while on holiday. But his doctor didn't
like the look of him and sent him for an immediate ultrasound.
By the end of the day, he had been diagnosed with disseminated
bowel cancer. He tolerated the first rounds of chemotherapy poorly
and despite being given other options he decided they would
not make a substantial difference in his case and opted for palliative care.

Last week, his community nurse urged him to spend some time
in hospice for respite and adjustment of his painkillers. He hesitated
at first but then, feeling sorry for his wife and family, who were keeping an anxious watch over him day and night, he agreed. In hospice,
he discovered that some of his assumptions had been wrong and
the team did manage to fine-tune his pain relief so that it hurt to
a lesser extent. But he missed home, his bed and his ten-year-old
golden retriever, and had no intention of giving the hospice a blank
order to continue to keep him there. He had accepted from the
start that nobody would be able to perfect the many nuances of
comfort care and, to his thinking, being pain-free for half the day
on most days was a worthy goal.

But as he was about to be discharged, he heard a crack as his
legs crumpled underneath him. It took all his presence of mind to
push the alarm as he hit the bathroom floor. He was bundled off
to the emergency department of the local hospital to have a pin
placed in his badly fractured right hip.

'You should look at the X-rays – the femur was twisted at a ninety degree angle,' he said.

The operation itself went uneventfully. But in the week since, he has developed acute kidney and liver failure. He did not see the orthopaedic surgeon after the operation, and was in so much pain beforehand that he cannot remember if he ever met the man, so he did not feel as if he was missing out on his care by leaving the busy and uncomfortable orthopaedic ward to return to hospice.

I had met him only briefly when he fractured his hip. I gave way at the doorway of the hospice to the ambulance officers who were taking him to hospital. When he screamed in pain, I quickly signed an order for a higher dose of morphine. I notice in an instant now that the change in his condition is dramatic. Loose folds of skin hang limply from his frame and his hands shake perceptibly as he reaches for his eyeglasses. His metallic green walking frame, a constant presence of late, is gone. In its place there are many more flowers, whose bright colours do little to obscure the bleakness of his outlook.

He breaks into my reverie. 'Can I trouble you for a bottle?'

'Yes, of course.' I want to be useful before he quizzes me on his condition.

We both forget that he does not need a bottle because he has a catheter.

Once he realises this, I turn to face him and there is an awkward moment of silence between us. He is an eminent and, until recently, active physician with incalculable wisdom behind his eighty years. I am some fifty years his junior, my career gaping with inexperience, and I am suddenly not sure how to interact with him. I vaguely recollect listening to him lecture early in my medical training. But I had a few white-haired professors and I am sure that his physique all those years ago would have been very different from the broken body he now inhabits. By all accounts, he is still a scintillating academic and this is what worries me the most now as I stand before him. Will he interrogate me about the latest studies on bowel cancer even though he gave up on treatment himself? Does he wish to know the results of his blood tests, awful as they look? Does he realise how long he has, or will he ask me? What did his doctors tell him? I can find no documentation of such a conversation in the notes. I fear that, trapped in his hospice bed, he could spend all day testing my knowledge and gauging my opinion. I brace myself to be gentle but firm.

I suspect that like many other patients he will offer little resistance if I look busy and adhere to the predictable checklist.

I have covered his pain.

'Do you have nausea?'

'Sometimes. But they give me stuff for it.'

'As you know, morphine can constipate. How are your bowels doing?'

'Oh gosh! Don't ask. After five days, I went today. This in itself makes it a good day.' He sighs. 'It's not fair, is it?'

I grumble it's unfair when the last can of drink has not been replaced in the fridge on a hot day. Or when there is pouring rain and someone sneaks into the last remaining parking spot. An eminent doctor and academic reduced to celebrating the opening of his bowels – is there a word to do justice to this?

'And how are your spirits holding up?'

Because I would be miserable, I think. Miserable that my life, spent warding off illness in others, had to culminate in this. Cheated that the end was so protracted, painful and, to be frank, a great big mess.

'My spirits? Thank you for asking, my dear. I think I just keep cycling through the seven stages of grief like one of those experimental rats!'

He laughs appreciatively at his own joke and I join in. And I am suddenly reminded of where else I have met him. He is a psychiatrist and I heard him as a guest speaker at a seminar many years ago on cancer and grief. He spoke eloquently and persuasively about the need to screen cancer patients for signs of depression, which was more prevalent than commonly perceived, illustrating his talk with some poignant recollections from his long career.

Then he falls silent and I think that this is my opportunity to leave. But somehow, it does not seem right to go now. Within him, I sense a willingness, if not eagerness, to talk and within myself a desire, or perhaps an obligation, to listen. I hope that he has fewer questions and more witty observations.

As I pull up a chair, he smiles invitingly.

'Doctor —,' I start.

He holds up his hands momentarily. 'Please, *you* are the doctor. I am only a patient in your hands.'

'Don't you want me to call you doctor?' I ask, genuinely surprised. The last thing I want to do is rob him of the deference his position deserves.

He shakes his head and grimaces. 'After my liver ultrasound, I was waiting for my wife when a young lady came into the waiting room waving a sheet of paper at me saying this was going to take longer than they thought. The report said "the liver is replaced with innumerable metastases". I was looking forward to returning to work and hadn't even remotely suspected I had cancer – the realisation felt like a guillotine.' His eyes cloud at the recollection. 'Who receives a diagnosis in the waiting room? Is that how you do things these days? Throw the report at the patient? At least I knew what it said!'

'That would have been difficult,' I sympathise, privately aghast at the insensitivity. 'Did she think you might want to know quickly because you are a doctor?'

His eyes seek me out before he replies evenly, 'Sometimes, doctors need doctors too.'

I instinctively wonder whether his uncharacteristic admission is borne of weakness or truth as it dawns on me that I cannot recall ever hearing this message outside of a well-meaning lecture in medical school.

Between eager sips of water, his words tumble out urgently.

'When I broke my femur, I was in pain and very upset at what it prognosticated. Every doctor knows that a fractured hip in an old man with cancer is the beginning of the end. The treating teams followed the checklist – drugs for pain, daily X-rays for check-ups because the surgeon was worried that the pin had moved, but there was a maddening blindness to my needs as a human being. At last count, I had a surgeon, two physicians, an anaesthetist, a social worker, multiple nurses and a physiotherapist seeing me. They checked every list that they carried, yet it never felt like anyone actually cared. As I lay in bed, I thought that if I were able, I would rather kill myself than suffer the indignity of being a mere object.'

He is unforgiving in his assessment of the medical system that strived to fix him but never succeeded in identifying his real needs. His voice drops and he looks momentarily asleep, as if he hadn't spoken at all. As I absorb the weight of his words, he is awake again.

'I felt no warmth or eye contact, no real connection during all my time at the hospital. And here's the funny thing. When I told the charge nurse how I felt, it was the only time she looked me in the eye and asked if I was okay. Then she called the psychiatrist!' He shakes his head. 'He was a nice chap, one of my early students.'

'And did he have anything to say?'

'He agreed with me that this sort of treatment was enough to precipitate a feeling of depression.'

Sensing I will be here for some time, I place his file by his feet.

It is overflowing with notes, investigations and recommendations. Spotting the bulging notes, he says exasperatedly, 'Why did the hospital need to do bloods every day? What's the point?'

It takes personal experience to understand the pain we inflict on patients by the mere stroke of a pen. I remember well my feeling of helplessness in hospital when I didn't have a say in being bled for tests that didn't make a difference.

'Do you want to know what they show?' I enquire. My fingers are ready to flick to the page, my lips eager to combat his many existential questions with but one concrete answer.

The exasperation returns to his face. 'No, no. I *know* I am dying. Even though I am a psychiatrist, I know what having liver and renal failure entails. Just because I understand the numbers doesn't mean I *need* to know them.'

I sit back, contrite at my misplaced alacrity to heal his wounds with a band-aid solution. I revolt against a sudden suspicion that this may be the only way I know.

'I just want to talk,' he says, like a firm but kind teacher. 'It's what I have done all my life with my patients, so humour me.'

'I am listening,' I promise, like a chastised student.

So steering away from all medical topics we talk about his grandchildren, especially the one with Down syndrome who has done him proud by growing up into a gentle young man. His youngest daughter had casually sought his advice about prenatal testing and he had advised against taking the risk of amniocentesis as she was still young and had two healthy children. There were some stressful years before his grandson's learning difficulties were attributed to Down syndrome. He recalls the many years of self-blame before his daughter helped him come to terms with the situation that no one could have foreseen. 'William started off at a remedial school and now goes to his local high school where he is in the top band

of students. I feel as if God has granted me a reprieve.' His pride
and wonderment are obvious as he points to a picture of a handsome William, poised amidst his ten other grandchildren from
four daughters.

He cries about his wife's impending widowhood but expresses
relief that the mortgage on their house is paid. They had been out
walking their sleepless child in the stroller when they strayed into
an expensive neighbourhood.

'It was the most dilapidated house in the best street.'

The agent talked them into the wise investment although the
fledgling psychiatrist and his wife wondered how they would meet
the repayments that sounded exorbitant fifty years ago. The young
couple renovated the house in stages, between children, transform-
ing it into their most coveted asset.

'I think I finally have the bank's permission to die!' he quips.
I can imagine him being entertaining and popular company and
feel sad I didn't know him in his heyday.

As if randomly leafing through his memories, he asks, 'When
you finished training, how did you go about finding a job?'

Warming to him, I grin.

'The normal way. I scoured the newspapers for job vacancies,
made many phone calls which translated into a few interviews and
one job. But I bet your story is more interesting!'

'When I finished psychiatry training, I was wondering what kind
of a job to take. One day, I heard a knock on the front door and
there was a man asking if I would consider a hospital appointment.
They really needed psychiatrists and my wife said yes and that was
that. I guess it's a bit harder these days.' There is a brief twinkle in
his jaundiced eyes. His stories are from a bygone era.

He expresses regret and frustration at the fracture that made
him spend an emotionally taxing week in hospital but returns to

focus on his positive experience at the hospice. He explains that he never felt a sense of entitlement from the establishment he had served for half a century but neither did he expect abandonment during his time of need. Now tiring, he berates modern medicine for becoming so enraptured with cure that it often denies care. Several times, I open my mouth to speak but his compelling words return me to silence. There is no bitterness in them, only sound reflection, gravity and lessons never so eloquently taught. It is just like the man I heard speak all those years ago, I think, regretting that his last meaningful contribution to medicine is to a private audience of one.

Soon the hour has passed and my hand has grown warm in his. His eyelids flutter under the weight of a heavy sleep, brought about by the unfiltered levels of toxins in his bloodstream. I realise how unfounded my fears were about treating another doctor at the end of life. While I feared the onslaught of medical questions, all he wanted was to be a patient, no different from others, equal in their need for comfort, hope and understanding, delivered not as an optional extra but as a core component of medical care. The difference perhaps lies in his ability to bravely express a sentiment that many others suppress for fear of alienating their doctors.

'Maybe, if it's okay with you, I could write about your experience one day. We could all learn something from it.'

He rouses himself temporarily and looks at me with interest.

'Do you write?'

'When I am moved. Your story is like that.'

'Get me a piece of paper, young lady. You will need consent.' For a fleeting moment, he looks like the interested and engaged professor he must have been.

I hand him a blank sheet and watch in amazement as he picks up his fountain pen, then his glasses, ceremonially adjusting them on his nose before proceeding to write out his consent in clear, bold letters. You have to study it closely to notice that the script wavers a little toward the end, before finishing in a subtle smudge as I rescue the pen falling out of his weak hand.

'Thank you,' I say.

But he has fallen asleep. I rise from my chair to leave, taking care this time to be quiet. In my anxiety to treat him differently, I almost did him a disservice. Fortunately, the teacher in him had the last word.

7

◇

I'm afraid it's bad news

The sun dawns lazily on a wintry morning. Beads of frost sparkle against alert blades of lush green grass; the sky is a blanket of startling blue. I awake with a delicious sense of anticipation.

I am five months pregnant. In a few hours, the twins I am carrying will appear live on an ultrasound screen. So far they have been only specks, their parts not identifiable despite the assiduous attempts of the technician. I have listened to their hearts beat, always racing each other to an imagined finish line. Just lately, I have noticed small movements, their attempts to communicate from within. Every day, I wait for their arrival which cannot come soon enough. I feel nervous, excited, giddy and lucky all at the same time as I wait to watch their transformation from amorphous masses to wondrous bodies.

My husband and I returned three days ago from an academic sojourn in the United States. Also a doctor, he gained business credentials while I used my Fulbright Award to complete a fellowship in medical ethics at the University of Chicago. He has a job interview this morning. I start work as a qualified specialist after the weekend. The time away has allowed extended soul-searching about exactly what sort of an oncologist I want to be; I am somewhat nervous but satisfied at an achievement that had seemed simply beyond imagination more than a decade ago, when I listened wide-eyed to the dean's welcoming lecture to first-year medical students. We are searching for a house that will accommodate our twins, jobs that will grant us flexibility. Our belongings lie scattered in borrowed space. Papers fly everywhere, the phone rings insistently and we survey the thick layers of dust that have gathered atop our carefully stored furniture. Nothing except our happiness seems assured. Like many of our friends, we deferred parenthood to meet the demands of medical training. Now, a new frontier in life can finally open.

Thus far, I have defied all the usual irritants of pregnancy. My obstetrician in the United States was happy with my progress; when I left, I promised to be in touch with her once the twins she had discovered entered the world. I can still recall the expression on her face as she looked at the ultrasound screen for the first time. She must have seen many sets of twins during her time, yet the wonder of discovering a twin pregnancy still enthralled her. In that small dark room, as she printed out nondescript images, we were all beaming at our secret, shared for the moment only by the three of us.

Having moved back to Australia, this is my first ultrasound before seeing my new obstetrician. I convince my husband to concentrate on his job interview, vowing to bring back pictures of the twins from what, after all, is going to be a quick, routine scan. He reluctantly agrees.

The hospital where I have spent all of my days as a medical student and doctor stands bathed in sunlight, imposing yet reassuring. In the short walk to ultrasound, I pause several times to greet friends and colleagues hurrying about their routine. My happiness is infectious. Once I arrive, I am led straight into the ultrasound room where a doctor waits. He welcomes me pleasantly and gets started. We don't know each other. The momentary tingle of the cold gel on my skin gives way to a thrill as the screen comes alive. Recognisable arms wave wildly, first two, then four. Legs stretch out of their curled comfort into a dark cushion of fluid. Two faces become apparent. Do they bear an expression or is it merely my imagination? As the doctor performs his task attentively, I relax and watch the twins float inside me, my heart periodically bursting into a private ecstasy. I make polite conversation with him although I would be content to say nothing and feel everything. As we talk, his genial face suddenly registers concern and although he turns his face sideways, I have caught the look. He pushes the ultrasound probe a little deeper. Uncomfortable, I hold my tongue to concentrate on reading his expression. I am sure he will find whatever he is looking for and I try to relax and sink back into the bed to help him. Feeling a sudden urge to go to the bathroom, I force myself to wonder about my husband's interview.

He grimaces and suddenly it seems as if his easy confidence has evaporated.

'Is everything okay?' I ask.

The articulate doctor mumbles unintelligibly. This is my second warning sign.

'Is it serious?'

'Uh, I need to talk to your obstetrician first.'

He bolts out of the door before I can open my mouth. I lie on the narrow bed, clutching the naked steel frame my fingers have wrapped themselves around. The television screen, which moments ago had lit up with the images of twins, blinks in confusion before fading to nothing. I fix my stare on the screen to force it to live again. The dark, sterile room spins around me, silent and foreboding. I clutch my abdomen involuntarily to guard the precious cargo within. Then, I wait the longest wait of my life. I strain my ears to listen through the closed door but can make out nothing of the muted conversation. I tap my foot anxiously against the edge of the bed.

He returns and shuts the door behind him. Does he wear a sense of resignation or is it my mind concocting the worst?

'We need to talk,' he says in a sombre tone. I hurriedly get dressed and follow him from the ultrasound room, along the corridor to his office.

'Can I get you some coffee?'

'No.'

'Do you want to call your husband?'

'He is in an interview. I don't know where to find him.'

'Should we wait?'

I am overcome by suspense and anxiety. 'No, you can tell me.'

His secretary looks on sympathetically, falling discreetly behind us.

In his small windowless office, he distractedly shoves a pile of paper away from the desk and pulls out a chair for me. Then he changes his mind and gives me his own padded one. I observe wryly that not too many patients would need to sit down in his room afterwards, as they would leave after having their scan.

'I am afraid it's bad news.'

My heart explodes. I don't know how but I know what he's going to tell me, I just know. I recognise the look on his face. He is behaving in a manner that I have used only too frequently when delivering bad news to my own patients. The harder the news, the longer the prologue. Oh, how many times have I sung the same melody from the doctors' song sheet?

Turning a blank piece of paper towards me, he sketches a picture of a pregnant uterus. Blood vessels in red and blue criss-cross between the twins. My mind seems possessed by a preternatural cool as I say firmly, 'I want you to tell me the truth.'

Even as I ask him this, my heart thumps with the fear that a request for the truth means different things to different doctors. Will he tell me exactly what he knows or will he send me for more tests to more doctors? Will he be completely honest or hide behind a wall of words?

He rubs his forehead. 'The twins are very, very sick. They have a rare condition called twin to twin transfusion syndrome.'

The tears feel like crystals grating behind my eyes. 'Are they dying?'

'Yes,' he replies sadly.

My first thought goes to my husband, probably discussing impending fatherhood now that the official interview must be over.

'When will they die?'

'I can't say for sure but probably soon.'

'Is there a chance of saving one?'

'I don't like the odds.'

'Are you sure?'

'I am sorry.'

'I appreciate your frankness. It's not your fault. Do you need this room back?' How ridiculous that I feel duty-bound to be nice to the man who has just told me the worst news of my life.

I look up from the picture he has drawn to find him blinking away a few tears. In that instant, we are connected – a mature parent who feels the pain of the would-be parent.

He asks again whether I want my husband present. I call but he is not home yet. Determinedly, I tell the doctor to go ahead with the amniocentesis. I return to the room where the secretary silently assists me. Awkwardness envelops us – her regular job is to schedule his appointments, not help patients deal with bad news. The long, cold needle jabs my abdomen. I, who hate needles, feel nothing.

'What do I do now?' I ask mechanically.

'I would like you to have a second ultrasound tonight, with a newer machine,' he answers. 'I want some experts to have a look at the pictures.' He thoughtfully avoids any other mention of the twins. In a stunned daze, I gather my belongings.

I drive home, possessed by ice-cold fury, unable to follow the thread of any particular thought. I politely give way to traffic, even waving through a tentative old lady. I take the long route to the borrowed space we call home, wondering how I will tell my husband. When he greets me excitedly at the door, I take out the crumpled sheet of paper with the obstetrician's scribbles on it and, like an impassive teacher, I inform the father of my children that we will not see them alive. He is even more bewildered than I am, partly because he does not have a kind doctor at his side. We get in the car and drive across town for the second ultrasound.

We wait for all the scheduled patients to leave, hiding resolutely behind the newspaper. Finally, it is my turn. The same doctor greets me and leads me into a well-appointed room, different to the one this morning. The bed doesn't creak as much and the ultrasound machinery looks more sophisticated. Pictures of his children adorn the mantelpiece. We go through the same routine. He seems more tense now and concentrates on bringing the twins up on the screen. Another obstetrician arrives. After a wordless nod, he heads straight to peer at the screen, awash with images, numbers and sounds. He confirms his colleague's suspicion of the anomaly and leaves in silence. Outside, night has fallen. Peak-hour traffic is building. Our hopes are failing.

'I have called the paediatric cardiologist in,' the doctor says. 'He called to say he was stuck in traffic.'

Through our sadness, we realise the enormous favour he has done us by summoning a cardiologist on a Friday night. When the cardiologist arrives he immediately recognises my husband, who had once been his intern. The mood of the room changes instantly, from an inconvenient Friday night call-out to helping a distressed colleague. He is one of the best paediatricians in town. Placing one hand on top of the screen to move it around, he gives us a simple tutorial on the physiology of hearts dying in real time. One heart is overloaded with fluid, the second is parched. Inextricably linked, they are both destined to fail. He points to their sluggish beat, the signature of their silent struggle.

'Are they dying?'

'Yes. This is terrible. I am so sorry.'

'Thank you for doing this on a Friday night.'

I can't help but note the veneer of politeness that we doctors maintain in the face of immense loss. There are no tears, no hysterics, just an extremely civil exchange of views. It leaves me wondering how and when we develop a different emotional response to tragedy.

I lie in a hospital bed too bewildered to talk, too tired to cry. I sink in and out of sedation, catching drifts of conversations between the nurses and my husband. Drips, catheters, residents – the daily substrate of my professional life intrudes into the personal. The morning rounds team hovers outside my room, its discreet exchange beyond my earshot and caring.

The induced labour is long and painful, something I would have endured gratefully for a different outcome. The twins, in life and death, defy norms. I remember a saying commonly tossed around that doctors attract more than their share of unusual medical diagnoses. I lie there, wishing I was normal, boring. I shake violently from a fever and feel so dry that I could drink a river. Everyone is gentle, nice and quiet. I feel vulnerable, cheated and sad.

The odds continue against me as hours later I am wheeled to the operating theatre. I have seen this room a hundred times but never its ceiling. Strangers in green gowns and masks assure me that I am in good hands. Without my contact lenses, their faces are blurred. Half-sedated, I cannot fully comprehend them. All I know is that the twins are dead but I need a procedure to make sure that they have been fully extruded. A young anaesthetics fellow talks about intubation, reassuring me that it won't be for long. Something within me gives and I refuse to consent. I want her to use my existing epidural instead of putting a breathing tube down my throat and rendering me unconscious. I feel terrified about a further lack of control but I am also furious that I, who have helped so many patients to good outcomes, have this to endure. I feel emotionally akin to a toddler having a tantrum. The anaesthetist is clearly annoyed at my perceived obstruction.

'Why don't you want to be intubated?' she asks, casting me as yet another difficult patient wanting to play doctor.

The cold, narrow bed can barely fit my frame. Anaesthetists attack each arm, patting veins into submission. Burly men move to the foot of the bed, peeling off the thin sheet that covers my naked legs. Machines beep. I hear the hiss of oxygen. I want to explain that the reason I don't want to be intubated is because the thought of going to sleep terrifies me. I am afraid that after losing my pregnancy, there is more shock in store for me when I wake up. From the minute my routine ultrasound began, I have had all my control snatched away and I don't want her to deprive me of the ultimate control, my sentience. But I am too tired to form my words properly and am scared that no one will listen. Just then, the obstetrician arrives. The epidural stays. It is a minor victory that fills me with untold relief.

The procedure finished, I return to the delivery suite. The nurses sensitively decide not to transfer me to the ward for new mothers. Soft music wafts through the walls. A young nurse arrives on duty. 'It's busy,' she says cheerily. 'They are having twins next door.' Instantly recognising her mistake, she apologises profusely before staying out of my room for the remainder of the shift.

Due to the effect of the epidural, I cannot feel my legs the entire night. I keep asking my husband to check that they are there, that one foot has not climbed on another. Although I know it is ludicrous, I worry that pressure sores will appear on my heels in a few hours. I spend the whole night staring at the ceiling in the dark. The twins are lost but I want my legs back. I just want to feel whole again, I pray. As dawn breaks, there is a sudden twitch in my legs. Then, as if at a stroke of magic, sensation floods my legs. 'I can move my legs!' I exclaim, jiggling them up and down in bed. It is amazing how wonderful a small mercy feels after a large loss.

At some point, I am asked whether I want to see the twins. I decline. There has never been any question in my mind that I did not want to begin my memory of parenthood with the sight of death. My husband decides otherwise. In the room, he looks at them for a while and whispers a tearful goodbye. They are wheeled out. Our hearts are breaking. The finality of our loss is indescribable.

The next day, I decide to go home, guilty at occupying a bed. All doctors are acutely aware of the shortage of beds and I feel duty-bound to treat my own workplace fairly. I also know that a few extra days in hospital is not the answer for me. As my husband helps me pack my belongings, the social worker enters discreetly. He is tentative, just out of training. He takes a full history from me the way he has been taught. My husband signals that we don't need him but he is so earnest that I feel compelled to let him talk for an hour.

I leave the building through a side exit in the early hours of the morning. A nurse wheels me out and helps me into the car.

'You take care,' she says. 'I know what it feels like, but I promise you, it will get better.' Her spontaneous kindness threatens to bring tears to my eyes, but we hastily say goodbye.

In the aftermath of the tragedy, my husband and I read and re-read the literature on twin to twin transfusion syndrome. I blame myself, he seeks answers. I question my faith and we both shed defeated tears. Calls of sympathy and expressions of helplessness pour in like an avalanche. There is also plenty of conjecture. Was it something I ate? Was it an infection? Did someone put a curse on me? We sidestep the comments, our combined medical training giving us strength. I avoid looking in the mirror until it no longer reflects a pregnant abdomen. I ignore a follow-up appointment with the obstetrician, not having anything to discuss and loath to sit in a waiting room with expectant mothers. As soon as I am able, I resume long walks. Slowly, as the pain of exercise subsides, I start to think about my life again. I become despondent quickly and then angry and resentful. But I eventually resurface. It seems like a tedious process. Surrounded by a sea of people, I have never felt so alone.

In the next few months, as the overt reminders of pregnancy fade, small incidents begin to form the scaffolding on which I rebuild myself. First, I recover physically, and for the first time fully appreciate what it is like being weak, unable to do the things one takes for granted. I cry with relief the first time I can walk around the local park without pain. I sink into the grass in disbelief the first time I can run. It is sad that it takes a period of disability to make you appreciate the able body.

Then, letters start to flow in from far-flung places where I have volunteered or lived. While some express shock at the news, many more treat it with resignation, even acceptance. I am initially puzzled but soon realise that in the countries from where these letters arrive, people are used to the grim statistics of infant and maternal mortality, much of which is preventable. Many of those who have written have lost their parent or child under even more horrific circumstances. I hear from mothers I met while volunteering in the Maldives, mothers who watched their children swept away by the gargantuan waves of the tsunami. A little boy who saw his baby sister drown in the tsunami sends me a picture. A friend from India writes. Her sister gave birth to a full-term baby who was stillborn because the only obstetrician in town went away for two days. Another, while expressing remorse, writes about her father dying a painful death from throat cancer. There is no cancer specialist in the entire region. These are realities from which we in the rich world are largely shielded. I feel very grateful that my care took place in a world-class facility; skilled experts could not erase my trauma but did all they could to cushion it. When I venture out to work again, I am showered with kindness, concern and offers of assistance, more than many others could hope for.

And slowly but surely, I begin to place my experience in some perspective. The perspective does not diminish my own loss but helps me view it through a larger prism of understanding. Sometimes, there really are no plausible answers to the fundamental question, 'Why me?'

I find myself shaken from complacency and at a turning point. Will I allow myself to be embittered and tainted by the experience or can I salvage some lessons to inform the rest of my career? I have witnessed enough tragedies unfold, treated enough hapless victims of preventable diseases and experienced enough deficiencies in basic health care, both here and abroad, that it would seem an injustice to do any less.

I wonder if my experience will make me listen more closely to my patients. Will I sit down at their bedside instead of hovering over them, pronouncing on their illness? Will I remember to feel their pulse despite the display of the monitor, now that I know that a gentle touch can be as therapeutic as the strongest medicine? Will I teach my residents that sophisticated tests are not a substitute for compassionate care and that when a patient expresses concern over a procedure, it is important to ask why instead of saying 'don't worry'?

Will I still roll my eyes at those who fail to keep the occasional appointment? In the past I assumed they simply had no regard for how busy doctors are but now I know that sometimes patients avoid doctors for the reminders they bring of illness and dependence. Will it take me long to forget that no aspect of a patient's presentation is uninteresting or commonplace, that to each individual, an illness feels like it has never quite struck someone else in the same way?

I want to think that I will perform my duty as a physician by treating not only the disease but the whole patient. I wish that it had not required a personal experience to determine the course of a profession, but if my loss achieves this, it will not have been all in vain.

8

◇

I am going to beat this

If doctors are allowed to confess to favourites, then Irma would be my clear choice, for the simple reason that when I see Irma, she cheers me up within a few minutes of our meeting. For the rest of the time she spends in my office, she effortlessly drives away the sombreness that forms an unavoidable part of the day-to-day work of being an oncologist. Her sheer zest for the concept of a well-led life and joy in the living of it makes me rejoice and restores my sometimes-wavering faith in the redemptive power of modern medicine.

Today, I can see her tucked away in her usual corner of the waiting area. I wave to her as I usher in other patients and relatives. She is as punctual as I am delayed in seeing her on the majority of her visits. But it is just like her to wave my apology away as she laughs at the half-eaten apple peeping out from behind my computer. 'It's not as if you are having a five-course lunch in here, darling! I know how hard you all work.'

There are days when I feel I could exchange all my patients for one encounter with Irma, not because I care any less about them but because she has that rare knack of making me temporarily put aside my responsibilities and see the world through a different set of eyes. Her observations about life are incisive, her relish for seemingly ordinary events like a road clear of traffic or a break of brilliant sunshine is delightful, but it is her almost lustful pleasure in being alive that is palpable and downright infectious. Every doctor needs a patient like Irma.

It is close to two years ago now, but the details of Irma's remarkable journey are clear in my mind. I am running late for a meeting and scan the list of unseen patients to select someone who is likely to be quick. A cursory flick through Irma's thin file assures me that she fits the bill. She is in her late sixties and, having been well all her life, recently presented to the emergency department with florid jaundice that her son noted on his return from a holiday. As every medical student knows, painless jaundice in an adult is cancer until proven otherwise. A CT scan revealed the suspected cancer occupying and blocking a large section of her bile duct. Irma was admitted to hospital, where she underwent a number of tests to confirm the diagnosis. A metal stent was placed in the bile duct with rapid resolution of the jaundice. The discharge summary tersely states her case: 'Previously well elderly lady with biliary cancer, not operable due to size and position. For oncology review and palliative care. Patient informed of poor outlook.'

As I walk up to the waiting room with Irma's file, I feel grateful that someone has taken care of the details. It is not uncommon for patients to walk into my office not quite sure why they are there. It falls to me to confirm that the euphemisms of mass, lump, abnormal cells and shadow that they have been hearing all along confirm their worst fear of a cancer diagnosis. And along with my pronouncement, I watch the last vestiges of hope come to a crash, the play of a hundred different emotions on a blanched face as the shoulders sink and moisture glazes the eyes of even the most hardened individual. If it were not for the palpable and transferable dread of the moment, it would be almost reverential to be in it. No matter how many times I do this particular task, it never feels easy or comfortable – and nor should it be. Nevertheless, I am grateful for someone else to have shouldered the burden this time.

The first time I call out Irma's name she answers from a corner. Quickly gathering up her bag and X-rays, she makes for my office. She is slightly built and has shoulder-length greying hair. A stray strand skims her right eyebrow. Her attire is simple; old but neat. There is not a button out of place or a crease on her blouse or skirt. Her face is devoid of makeup but her warm smile seeps into all the wrinkles, lighting it up effortlessly. Wondering what fears hide beneath, I invite her to sit down and tell me all she knows about her cancer. A sneaked look at my watch tells me I have twenty minutes with her. I am sure that will be enough for the 'no cure but comfort' talk, as a colleague wryly puts it.

'I will give you plenty of time to ask me questions but I want to hear your side first,' I say.

She shrugs her petite shoulders. 'All they have told me is that I have a tumor in the bile duct and I have six months maximum.'

'I see.' I didn't expect her to encapsulate her predicament so neatly in one sentence.

'But I tell you, I am going to beat this, I am!'

I don't hear this vow as often as I would like; however, I sense her chance of making good on it is bleak.

But her eyes narrow with determination and her small frame assumes a fierce and almost predatory stance. 'I don't know what sort of doctors they make that one of them could look me in the eye and say, "You'd better just go home and be in peace. There's nothing anybody can do."' Still affected by the recollection, she pauses and reaches out for a tissue to wipe her nose. 'You would think he'd never had a family member who was sick.'

'I am sorry,' I offer, uncomfortable with the insensitivity she describes. But patients frequently recollect and reinterpret the worst of what they are told, as I know all too well from my own experience, so I press on.

'Did anyone give you other advice?'

'The surgeon came at about six o'clock one morning, when I was fast asleep. I was still opening my eyes and he mumbled something about this being a bad cancer that he could not operate on. I was trying to think of some questions but he said his assistant would come by later. Since then, I seemed to see a different doctor every day until they said I was ready to go home because my jaundice was gone. I insisted that I would like to see a cancer specialist and they made me an appointment but also told me not to expect too much.'

'I am sorry you have had such a rough time.'

She looks only slightly mollified and studies my face hopefully.

'Let's have a look at your films.' I flick on the light switch to study her CT scan. I don't need the report to spot the ominous mass embedded in her liver. Enfolding major blood vessels, it looks impossible to remove, even to my non-surgical eye.

'Have you seen the scan?' I ask. Like many patients, she is interested and comes up behind me. I point to it with the tip of my pen.

'That looks big.'

We proceed to the examination table, where I find her jaundice resolved and her health otherwise perfect. It is when we are seated again I must voice the opinion that I have already formed. I want to tell her that as fit and well as she looks today, I too am certain that her lease on life is tentative. Perhaps I would use different words to say so but I believe that treatment in this case may prove futile and full of unwanted side effects that would make a liability of the remainder of her life. Inwardly, I feel that guiding her towards palliative care is the appropriate move. But hoping to find a lead from her, I listen to what else she has to say.

'What I don't understand is why anyone would give up so easily. In my life, I have fled war, divorced an alcoholic husband and brought up a child on my own. Every time people have said life is bad I have fought hard and won. So I am not going to let anyone tell me this time is different. I am going to do whatever I can to beat it and then see what happens.'

Her short speech would sound desperately clichéd if it were not for the defiant blaze of conviction that accompanies it. Even for one who listens to a few such predictions every day, I cannot help but feel swept up by the wings of her hope. I excuse myself as I leave the room to postpone my next meeting. Irma is going to take more than twenty minutes.

'Irma, I have to tell you that although cancer treatments have progressed, biliary cancer is still a hard one. We have limited options.' I discuss the available chemotherapy and its side effects and then spend equal time on supportive care measures such as pain relief and ongoing management of her jaundice if it worsens. I don't want to bias her or talk her out of treatment, but how does one draw the line between being biased and the good of the patient? When faced with tough choices, patients will often ask, 'What would you do if you were in my situation?' This can be a difficult question to answer and one that I try to avoid, because it is well known that doctors view the often small benefits of cancer therapy in a dimmer light than patients and state that they would forego standard treatment for certain cancers given present success rates. But these are hypothetical questions put to healthy doctors – no scientific study can ever really tap into the depth of dread and desperation when cancer strikes. Nevertheless, I wish Irma would ask for my recommendation. Instead, she has ears only for discussing her treatment.

'I am going to fight this,' she declares again. 'And I need your help.'

'Okay, Irma.' I realise that she will not accept anything short of treatment, and she is entitled to her hopes as much as I am entitled to my doubts. 'I will chat to some colleagues and treat you as best we can.'

'Thank you, doctor. You are the first person to listen to me. Don't worry, it will be okay.' She rises to gather her belongings and waves goodbye, the smile back on her face.

I shake my head at her unusual resolve, wondering whether it will assist her through the rest of her life or simply serve as a bigger let-down. But, keeping my word, I discuss her case with others. The next week, she convinces my colleague to add in some radiation to her treatment. He explains to her that the chances of remission are small and that of cure even smaller. But, like me, he is impressed by the strength of her will and agrees to do what he can.

The next time I see Irma, she has had the initial week of treatment.

'How are you doing?' I ask anxiously.

'Great, darling!' she exclaims. 'All the things you wrote down for me – nausea, vomiting, fatigue – I don't feel a thing!' Underneath her jacket, she pats the small pump that provides a continuous weekly infusion of chemotherapy. 'This is not a problem at all.' She beams at me. 'Thank you for arranging all this.'

Pleased and immensely relieved that she looks as sprightly as she does, I nevertheless feel obliged to add, 'Irma, these are early days. I hope all your treatment goes well.' If she senses the warning in my voice, she deftly ignores it. And so it is that week after week, for six weeks, she returns for a review, defying my prediction and coping admirably with the rigorous schedule of therapy.

'You do what you have to do,' she tells me. 'This is what was meant to happen to me, but I can choose how to deal with it.' Sometimes I cannot help thinking that she sounds like a self-help audio book, but it is hard not to marvel at her tenacity.

'I am very glad that you are coping so well,' I say to her. However, I am careful never to venture beyond what her keen ears must note are mere platitudes. But if she senses that I am not convinced her treatment will be worthwhile, she does not let it bother her. I am conscious that as her doctor I should not be the antidote to her enthusiasm, but to flame it would also gnaw at my conscience when I have seen far too many cases like hers end sadly.

After she has finished treatment, she comes to see me, her grin broader than ever. 'You know, the radiation doctor just did a scan and most of the tumour has gone!'

She hands me the films. As I put them up on the same screen I used when I first met her, I find myself hoping that she is right. And indeed she is! The large tumour that sullied the neat architecture of the area has shrunk to a nubbin, still visible but nowhere near as threatening as it had appeared before. I turn to Irma.

'Congratulations, Irma! That really is a great result!'

'I couldn't have done it without you. I brought you something,' she says next. Out of a bag, she withdraws a large cake, exquisitely frosted with the words 'thank you'. I am touched. Given the hundred doubts I have harboured all along, I find her gesture particularly generous and undeserved.

'You know, when I came here for the first time, I was terrified. And once you heard me out and gave me time, I just felt better knowing that someone had listened. I will never forget my first visit.'

'Irma, it's what they pay me to do!' I say with embarrassment. 'You deserve the credit!'

'How about we share it?' she suggests, with a laugh that seems open to believing in endless miracles. She gives me a hug and says, 'I better clear out! There are other people who need you more.'

In the almost two years since that conversation, Irma has returned regularly for reviews, which sometimes include blood tests and scans. On each occasion, I tell her that she looks remarkable and there is no sign of her tumour growing. It is only after I have told her this that her composure softens and she confesses she has not slept since the scan. Then she brings out her cake, a different one each time, each seemingly larger and more elaborate than the last. I whoop with amazement at her talent and she sits back to relish my genuine pleasure. Then, as if on cue, her phone rings. Winking at me, Irma answers it.

'Yes, darling,' she speaks into the phone. 'No, she said nothing to worry about. I would tell you . . . She is very busy, but I will ask her. Hold on a minute.' She shakes her head like a teenager in love.

I take the phone from her.

'Is the cake sweet enough, you reckon? I think she doesn't put enough sugar in!' a man bellows heartily down the line.

'I haven't tried it yet, but it looks delicious, thank you, James.'

'So tell me the truth. Is she okay?' His voice falls to a whisper. 'You know she wouldn't tell me even if something was wrong.'

'James, the scan is clear, the bloods look good. You can relax now.'

'Then what kind of cake do you want next time?' he laughs, the relief in his voice palpable.

I find this one of the most endearing routines of my day whenever I see Irma. Over time, I have come to know more about her. Once she knows that her results look good, she doesn't like to dwell on her disease anymore. I now know that she left her first husband soon after her son was born. The baby was just a year old, but she was determined to bring him up properly and so made this and other difficult decisions, including taking up a job to support her child. Although her family regularly prompted her to remarry, she firmly believed that any new husband would compete with her son for her affections, so she stayed single until her son finished university and got married himself. Irma married her long-time friend James eight years ago. Last year, James suffered a stroke that left him in need of help. She willingly accepted that her duty was to help him deal with his disability even as she monitored her own health. Theirs seems an easy and friendly relationship, built on mutual assistance and respect. James sometimes accompanies her to the consultations but prefers to sit outside.

'He is too nervous to come in first. But if you say it's good news, he will join me,' she explains.

Irma also talks lovingly about her grandchildren and how her love for her son is multiplied when she cares for his three children. Other times she tells me about her garden, which she has carefully tended over the years, and her walking group, which has stuck together for thirty years. As the fabric of her life emerges more fully, I find her to be one of the most adjusted and happy individuals I have ever met. And I look forward to peering through her eyes into life in all its glory.

Irma and I have never talked about her being cured because she recognises very well that the sword of recurrence will always hang over her. But it is how she treats whatever time she has left that is nothing short of inspiring. Without probably ever caring to make it her mission, she has succeeded in making me respect the power of self-belief. Irma was the only one who ever believed that she could beat her cancer. Her doctors, including me, found her resolve so infectious that we felt compelled to give her the benefit of the doubt.

I like to see Irma and be reminded that sometimes, doctors can get it wrong. Wrong as to how a disease will behave and wrong about how a patient will cope. It is not a reflection of the lack of skill but more a reminder of the diversity of nature, the reach of biology and the immeasurable contribution of individual traits such as confidence, faith and hope.

9

◇

Send me home

If you hear Alana's son tell the story of how it all began, you will laugh: he, with his eighteen years of accumulated wisdom; he with the immaculately disarrayed hair – a work of art made possible, his siblings would claim, by rising early and using hairspray often; he with the lately acquired nonchalance of adolescence, who is quick to whiff embarrassment, especially when dealt in the form of parental mishaps.

'So there we are in the fruit section and Mum says, "Get a few of these. We're running out of potatoes." The potatoes are all the way at the end of the aisle so I begin to walk there. And she shouts, "Jamie, sweetheart, I mean these potatoes." I turn around and she is holding up a rosy, red apple. So I say, "Do you want apples or potatoes, Mum?" She looks at what she is holding and says, "Sorry, apples, we need apples. Come and weigh some apples with me." So I shake my head and avoid looking around me as I walk back to Mum. She smiles and pretends nothing happened. I toss the apples in the trolley and move on with Mum.

'We get to the frozen section and I spot this girl I really like, who is shopping with her dad. I mean, I really, really like Ella. She's in the same year as me and I've been waiting for months to ask her to our formal. Ella is a really good artist and has won a couple of big competitions. She also does singing and ballet, everything that I'm not good at. Anyway, what I'm saying is that she's cool and nice and I like her a lot. I think you get the point. So I'm deciding whether to wave to Ella or just walk past, pretending I'm so absorbed in shopping I didn't even notice her, when Mum calls out, "Jamie, pumpkin, come over here."

'Pumpkin? My mother has never called me pumpkin in all the years I have been able to decipher what she is saying. So keeping one eye on Ella, I ignore the call, keep staring at the ice cream while inching away from my mum. But if you know my mum, you know she has a low opinion of discretion. So she shouts, "Jamie, pumpkin, do you think we should get apple pie for dessert?"

'Oh God! Ella turns her head towards me, and waves. "Hi James!"

'"Hi." I wave slowly, my horrified expression not meant for her but for my mother, who is holding a leg of lamb in her hand.

'"Yes, mum, that's fine." I smile, hoping that I've taught her well enough to tell my smiles apart, because this smile is supposed to say, "Mum, you are suffocating my budding lovelife."

'"This must be your mum. Hi! I'm Ella." We're all standing in front of the dessert section, doing the introductions, the true significance of the situation dawning on my mum, who is now trying to figure out how to impress with a leg of lamb at first glance. I nod exaggeratedly at Ella and her dad, we exchange some pleasantries that I don't have the heart to recall and, grabbing Mum by her free arm, I say, "Let's go. We have to hurry up for my piano practice."

'It's Ella's turn to be surprised. "I didn't know you played the piano," she exclaims. "Dear God," I think.

'Dear old Mum to the rescue this time: "Jamie is good at —"

'I practically push my mother out of the store before she is arrested for misrepresenting food items or her children's talents.

'In the car, I say, "Mum, OMG!"

'"What?" she asks, puzzled.

'"Oh my God!"

'"What happened, darling?"

'"Don't worry," I sigh, already ruing the briefest courtship in history.

'So that night at dinner, Dad asks what we did today, and I told everyone about going to the store with Mum. Mum says it didn't happen, my little brother and sister laugh their head off, but Dad, being a paramedic, gets a worried look on his face.

'"You should get your head scanned, honey," he says to Mum, eating the last of his soup.

'We all giggle. "You mean there's a scan to explain why parents are embarrassing?"

'"We'll see," says Dad, rubbing his own head.'

A CT scan confirmed Alana's husband's worst suspicion. A tumour lay in her brain, in the area associated with naming objects. The neurosurgeon said she was lucky the spot was easily accessible and she went into hospital to undergo surgery. Pathology revealed the tumour to be a secondary cancer but an exhaustive search for its origin proved futile.

She comes to see me after the neurosurgery, buoyed by the surgeon's pronouncement: 'He said he got it all! I owe him my life.'

'That's great, Alana!' I respond. 'I am pleased he was able to get it out.'

'But he said I would need radiation.'

'Yes, that's to prevent other tumours from appearing in the brain.'

'But the tumour was cut out, right, Mike?' she asks, looking to her husband for confirmation. 'Or am I forgetting that too?' She smiles wryly.

'You are right, darling.'

'What sort of side effects does radiation give you?'

'I am sure the radiation doctor will go through them in detail when you see him tomorrow.'

Alana teaches music at the local high school. She is particularly respected for her grasp of complicated scores, which she can apparently replay from memory. This makes me loath to tell her that radiation therapy can cause memory lapses. She is tall and has slender, agile fingers. I can picture her lost in her own world at the piano.

'So what happens now? Do I need to see you again? I know one of my friends sees her oncologist every year.'

It is the simple questions that break one's heart. I look at the woman seated before me, exuberant after successful surgery. She meets my eyes and smiles. I look at her husband. What does he know? He answers by avoiding my eyes.

I feel a familiar sense of exasperation. I want to ask her if the surgeon told her anything aside from the fact that he had done his job and obviously done it well. Did he not tell her that the tumour was a secondary deposit from an unknown primary cancer that still lurked in an organ, and we didn't know which one? Did he not even hint at the fact that this was not to be a casual visit but the beginning of a series of consultations as we waited for the cancer to emerge?

As I look at her guileless expression, I am suddenly reminded of a time very early in my training as an oncologist when I did rounds on postoperative neurosurgery patients. I would enter the ward each morning to be handed a list of patients by the neurosurgery resident, who would then promptly rush to assist with the theatre list. I would make my way through the patients, finding them in various states of sleep and wakefulness. Some patients would be propped up in bed eating breakfast while others, still attached to monitors and drips, waited to be sufficiently freed from wires to enable them to move. Part of their hair would be shaved to facilitate brain surgery, and bandages covered their sutured wounds. All but the sickest patients were to be found alone at that time of the morning, when visitors were discouraged to allow doctors to complete their rounds uninterrupted.

I will never forget the conversation with Mr Heatherton on one routine morning. I peered through a small chink in the green patterned curtains to check that he was awake before walking into his small cubicle. He was in his early fifties and recovering from neurosurgery performed two days earlier. The operation notes stated the diagnosis to be consistent with a glioblastoma, a uniformly fatal brain tumour that had a tendency to spread its tentacles into deep brain matter, making it impossible to remove completely. 'Major debulking performed but clearance not attempted due to risk of damage to vital functions including speech . . .' warned the notes. The progress notes since his operation consisted of not much more than brief remarks about his neurological function. He was recorded to be awake, cognitively intact and moving all his limbs. His speech was preserved, as were his other senses. I assumed that there was not much more to add in an otherwise healthy man who had never been to hospital before.

'Hello. I am one of the doctors from the cancer unit,' I introduced myself. He was working through his breakfast and looked up as I spoke, a serve of scrambled eggs heaped on his fork.

'Good, good thanks. Sorry, I missed who you said you are.'

'I am from oncology. Did your surgeon say to expect me?'

Mr Heatherton frowned. 'No, I haven't seen the surgeon since before the operation.'

'You may have seen someone from his team then . . .?' I prompted.

'I saw the resident yesterday,' he recalled.

'Did he say anything about the operation?'

'No. I asked him how it went but he didn't really say anything. He said he needed to replace my drip and was in a hurry.'

He took a mouthful of the egg and looked at me expectantly.

'So what do you know so far about your operation?'

'The nurse said that they had taken out a lump but they needed to wait for the final results to know whether it was cancerous. Why, do you know anything else?'

I closed my eyes for a second, paradoxically hoping that my doing so would prevent him from seeing the reaction on my face.

'I am afraid it was a brain tumour.'

'Oh, I knew it was a tumour, but we don't know whether it was a cancerous tumour.'

'Mr Heatherton, I am sorry to say that it was a glioblastoma, which is a type of brain cancer.'

His fork and knife fell to the floor with a clatter. In the silence that ensued, his easy expression underwent a rapid transformation and he turned ashen.

'Are you sure?'

'Yes. I am sorry.'

Following a few more seconds of silence, which shortchanged him but which was all I could afford on that busy morning, I continued my brief and talked him through the diagnosis, its implications and the treatment options. I kept my tone optimistic but my heart felt doleful, for I knew that I had lost him the moment I uttered the word 'cancer'.

'I am sorry this has arrived as a shock to you. I will check in again and also give your wife a call.'

He nodded distractedly, perhaps already lost in a world of reflection and calculation. He didn't really care what else I did.

Crestfallen, I walked out of his cubicle and repeated the encounter six more times. One was with a young man who had been stretchered in from the football field with seizures, another with an elderly Greek lady who did not speak much English but understood enough to be terrified, and another with a mother of two toddlers, who simply burst into tears and begged me to leave the room because she did not believe me. In each cubicle, I started off by assuming the patient knew at least the diagnosis, if not the treatment schedule, because the surgical team had called the oncology consult, after all. Before the operation, sophisticated scans had suggested that there was cancer. During the operation, the surgeon had seen and handled it. The surgeon's aide writing the notes had sketched a representation of the tumour and described it in writing. And sometimes, the pathologist had provided an on-the-spot assessment of the tissue sample. Yet the patient was the only person waiting on the formal printed pathology report to confirm the diagnosis of cancer.

In my first few days on the job, I attributed patients' surprise at the diagnosis of cancer to the usual factors: inattention, forgetfulness, denial. But it did not take long to trace the common thread between them – the surgeon was responsible only for the technical aspect of the operation, and the oncologist for everything else that followed. I could never understand why we allowed with such complacency, and even a sense of jocularity, that surgeons would be surgeons and that it was okay for many, if not all of them, to get away without communicating with their patients about their life-changing diagnosis.

These rounds were considered a necessary ritual for a trainee. Not once was I accompanied on these consultations by a mentor who would either object to this routine or at least reassure me that my discomfort was well-founded. By the time the consultant came around to hear me present the patients, some had been discharged and many were still recovering from the blow that my words had caused. The initial urgency of my own feelings had also died, leaving little room for meaningful debriefing. So what I learnt, absorbed or disavowed from these consultations was entirely up to me and, in many ways, the experience crystallised many of my ideas about how doctors should handle a diagnosis of cancer.

One day, after a particularly demanding and dispiriting series of consults, I asked the charge nurse why it was that surgeons did not talk to their patients.

'They are just not the sort, I guess. That's why they get people like you to come around,' she replied, her answer laced neither with irony nor any apparent frustration. In her twenty-five years of working with them, she had obviously made sense of a world to which I was a newcomer.

I remind myself that this is still the most complete answer I have received on the subject, as I return my attention to Alana. I find myself in a quandary about what to tell her. Like the surgeon, do I emphasise the obvious and congratulate her on the fact that he 'got it all'? Or do I temper the news by warning her that the primary tumour has yet to declare itself? A diagnosis of cancer brings such awesome and awful choices for the patient, and sometimes the doctor too. Should she be encouraged to believe that the only visible cancer in her body now lies bottled in a pathology jar, or should she be introduced to the fear that the true culprit is lurking in her body, avoiding detection, at least for now? If I were in her place, what would I want? I would want to know. Would the knowledge empower or stupefy me? I suspect the latter. But how can I be so presumptuous as to use my judgement as the standard by which to measure what is right for my patients? I fall back on the option that seems to work best most often. I ask the patient.

'Alana, the situation is not as straightforward as that, I am afraid. How much do you want to talk about today?'

She studies me. 'Don't mind my asking but do you have children?'

'Yes.' Since the loss of my twins during pregnancy, I have been blessed with two healthy children. My son is two and my daughter only a few months old.

'Okay. And I am assuming they are young,' she says, breathing out. 'Then you will know that my primary job is to protect them. So I want to know things but not to the extent that they can smell my fear.'

She has elegantly tossed the ball back into my court. After an involuntary thought of my children crosses my mind, I decide to deflect her from the imponderable to the tangible.

'What you need right now is radiotherapy. Have this and let us hope for the best. I have had some patients who have been long-term survivors after having a brain secondary treated. But we will need to keep a close eye on you.' I hope she and her husband register the word 'some', for this is what I most want them to heed.

She is pleased at the letting in of a glimmer of hope. She smiles readily, looks interested now, ready to join *this* category of patients. I imagine the conversation around her dinner table tonight, paraphrasing my words and hence my concerns: 'The doctor says not to worry. Lots of people in this situation do okay.' Will their mother's soothing misrepresentation of my fears serve to allay the anxieties of her children, even temporarily? I tell myself that if the answer is yes, I don't mind being misquoted.

'I will see you after radiotherapy, in a few weeks,' I conclude.

She leaves ahead of her husband to book the next appointment. Pretending to fumble with his jacket, he hangs back until she is well clear of my room.

'This is not going to go well, doc, is it?'

It is more a statement than a question.

'Mike, I wish I knew, but it really depends on what happens next.'

He looks unconvinced, so I hasten to reassure him, 'I am not hiding anything from you.'

Not for the first time, I wish there were better answers to some of the questions cancer patients ask. Sometimes, I find myself looking for a 'penicillin moment', when the ordering of a test or the prescription of a drug would answer a question definitively or eradicate a disease for good. But the world of oncology is nothing if not a continuum of worrisome questions to which there are maddeningly nuanced answers. Even the most optimistic pronouncements are chaperoned by disclaimers. 'You are okay for *now*'; 'We will do what we *can*'; 'The scans don't show anything *for the moment*.' The implied warning in all these statements is that circumstances can change, sometimes the day or the week after a reassuring visit. I realised the irony of the word 'relax' very early and stopped using it in conversations with my patients.

The next time I see Alana, she has completed whole-brain radiotherapy. Her face looks haggard despite her attempt to dress well and wear light makeup. Her skin has paled and she has lost some weight due to persistent nausea preventing her from eating. But there is also something else – a palpable sombreness to her expression, her previous confidence now stained by a new diffidence.

'How do you feel?' I ask.

'The radiotherapy was pretty taxing,' she offers. 'Apart from the nausea and headache, I still feel as if my head is swimming. I can't think straight and my concentration is poor. Does radiotherapy destroy your brain?' she enquires.

'I am sure these symptoms will settle down – you have only just finished treatment.'

'I am looking forward to being normal again.'

Out of her line of sight but directly in mine, her husband wrings his hands.

I prepare to speak but she steps in. 'Since I saw you, I have done a bit of research. I know that it's basically a waiting game from now on. Is that right?'

'Yes, we need to keep a close eye on you.'

She looks pensive and a film of tears forms over her eyes.

'This is going to be hard. Waiting is hard.'

What can I say to her about waiting? The times I have waited for answers have been nowhere as consequential. I remember waiting for news of my admission to medical school. I remember waiting on the phone to speak to the doctor when my mother developed septic shock on an international flight. I remember waiting at taxi ranks and airports, cursing the fog that prevents lift-off, but none of my experiences deserves mention in the same breath as the wait that faces her.

Any attempt to downplay the significance of her wait would sound like a platitude so I simply say to her, 'You are right.'

It takes another six months before her scans detect a tumour, hidden in the folds of her lung. It is only small, defying belief that it could be so rapacious as to spread not only to the brain but also to some other organs. There is an anticlimactic feel to my announcement.

Alana says, 'I feel relieved, like the intruder has been arrested.'

Mike says, 'Okay, so tell us how to treat this.'

I tell them that Alana's lung cancer is treatable, but not curable. I describe the available treatments and launch into an automatic rendition of what to expect from each, but I keep the description short. A respected oncologist once observed to me that even the seemingly well-prepared patient generally only recalls the first few minutes of a serious conversation. His observation has proved to be true in my experience and I try to give information in small packages. I am aware that whatever else I say, the take-home message for Alana and Mike is that she has terminal cancer. This is the fear that will gnaw at her and this is the clipped message that she will tearfully deliver to her friends and family.

'I am going to stop for a minute and give you time to ask me any questions you have. This is very difficult information to digest.'

She grips his hand tightly. I can tell from her expression that the questions in her mind are rushing faster than she can capture them in words. Most of us are bewildered by the choices we must make in the supermarket aisles, let alone those that literally concern life and death. I shuffle through paperwork while I wait. I have come to admire the sheer courage of patients who at this juncture manage to hold their emotions together and ask even one meaningful question, for I feel sure that I would find myself tongue-tied in a relationship as unequal as that between a doctor and a patient. As a doctor, I have seen metastatic lung cancer innumerable times, but this is Alana's first and only experience of having cancer.

Finally, she speaks. 'You know, I don't know what to ask. I mean, you need to know what you don't know in order to ask questions and I feel there is a lot I just don't know.' She stops suddenly in mock horror. 'Was I starting to sound like Donald Rumsfeld?'

We all laugh at the self-conscious reference. Then she says seriously, 'I'm sure I will have many questions along the way. But for now, I am going to concentrate on my kids and leave you to battle the cancer. Just do your best and keep me well through it.'

'But hang on!' I want to say. 'You can't leave me to make these decisions on your behalf. You need to understand the program, the side effects, and know what you are in for.'

'I'm not foolish,' she adds before I have had a chance to speak. 'For the time being, I just prefer not to know all the details if I don't need to. Then, there is less to keep from the children.' Stated such, her logic is faultless.

She starts chemotherapy. The side effects are immediate and overpowering. She is racked by nausea, vomiting and infections. When she comes in for review, she tells me that she has spent the past week in bed. I adjust her anti-nausea drugs, counsel her regarding diet and sleep, and encourage her to try a second round. The second week proves only marginally more tolerable. She looks spent.

'Do you think it is working?' She is asking for a reason to keep going.

'These are early days; you haven't even finished two whole cycles,' I say from behind her, glad she cannot see me as I listen to her lungs. I can't help but notice how her shoulderblades and ribs protrude. The skin on her arms sags and her voice sounds dull. Suddenly, my gut instinct says that she won't do well out of this. But gut instincts are just that, unsupported by objectivity, and I don't want to be overly pessimistic about her chances. I hover at her back a little longer than necessary. I cannot ban instinct, much in the same way as I cannot ban tears or sweat. And in fact, instinct is a crucial part of being a good doctor, for in denying instinct, one risks denying something fundamental about the art of being a doctor.

But then, I will myself to think of the patients who have defied not only my predictions but those of every other doctor who had expected them dead within six months.

'How do I sound?'

'Not bad,' I say. I don't know what to do. Should I stop her chemotherapy and ask her to have an early scan, effectively telling her I don't think her treatment is working? Or should I keep a lid on my dread and let her go through a few more weeks of therapy to make us both feel better? Would she rest easier for having given it her best shot or would she feel cheated that I let her endure those terrible toxicities in vain? And if by chance an early scan shows that she is responding, will she lose faith in me for my incorrect judgement? These questions quickly gather momentum and enormity in my mind. For a fleeting second, I wish the case away before realising that these are the very moments that distinguish a doctor's job as being a calling rather than a mere occupation; the day medicine ceases to toss up such live ethical dilemmas is the day I must re-evaluate my commitment to it.

'Alana, I need to discuss something with you.'

'Sure, are you not happy with things?'

I am impressed by her astuteness, no doubt sharpened by years of being a mother.

'I have nothing solid to back this up but I feel we should get another scan before you go on to another round of chemotherapy.'

She is puzzled. 'I thought you had explained that it's not useful to do scans too quickly as the tumour doesn't change so fast.'

I hate where this is going. 'I know, but I would feel better getting a scan.'

'Why, what have you found?' Her voice takes on a pleading tone.

'Nothing, but you don't look as well as I would like.' I, too, silently plead with her to indulge my worry and then prove it wrong.

'But chemo is supposed to make you sick! What do you expect?'

She is right. Suddenly feeling foolish for jumping to a conclusion, I am close to withdrawing my statement. But to my surprise, I say to her, 'It may turn out to be one of those scans to please the doctor rather than the patient, but I think you should have it.'

'Okay.'

I chastise myself for injecting fear and doubt into her, the opposite of what a good doctor is meant to do. As I hand her a request slip for a CT scan, I find myself hoping that we can both laugh at my exaggerated concern when she returns.

She comes back with her husband. The atmosphere is tense and, after greeting her, I take the scans from her hand. Putting the pictures up on the viewing screen, I ask her how she feels. 'I guess we will know soon,' she says.

The scan confirms my worst fears. The lung cancer has doubled in size and is now associated with numerous secondaries that have appeared in a matter of weeks. The innocuous-looking fluffy clouds of white will soon crowd out her normal lung. The spots in the liver have coalesced into large masses that could bleed or cause significant pain. Her bones look mottled.

My first reaction of feeling reprieved is rapidly followed by frustration and sadness for Alana. It takes all my grit to turn and face the couple.

'I am afraid the cancer looks worse. I don't think this chemotherapy is doing its job.'

Alana's face falls. 'I can't believe it – after all that sickness . . . What do we do now? Is there anything else?'

Grateful that she wants to talk about something that I can control, I tell her about other chemotherapy drugs.

'Second-line treatments are not usually known for providing a good response,' I counsel, 'but certainly, we can try something else, especially in someone who is young and fit like you.'

Her eyes take on a determined look again. 'I want to ask you a few questions and I would really like you to give me non-medical answers if you can.' By way of explanation, she says, 'I don't mean to be rude but I don't want to walk out of here wondering what you really meant.'

'I understand.' At least she knows what she wants, I tell myself.

'Is it very serious to have these results?'

'Yes.'

'Will more chemotherapy prolong my life?'

Patients ask this question in many forms and for a variety of reasons too, but I have always held that it must require extraordinary courage to frame it in a way that leaves no room for ambiguity.

'I don't think so.'

'Will more chemotherapy do anything, then?'

I hesitate before remembering her directive. 'Theoretically, it could shrink some spots and reduce a few symptoms, but I am not confident that it would do either in your case.' I also touch on some of the side effects of further chemotherapy, aware that to the patient who endures it, there must be no such thing as modest nausea or controllable diarrhoea.

'How long do I have?'

I knew it was coming. The oncologist's standard answer begins with, 'I am not exactly sure', followed by, 'Everyone is different . . .', and then by vague figures and hunches before concluding with, 'So in an individual case, it's very hard to predict . . .' I know because I follow minor variations of the routine every day.

Part of the reluctance of doctors to provide a prognosis stems from the fact that they are thought to be notoriously bad at it. Nothing saps one's confidence so much as a patient triumphantly returning for a five-year review, proclaiming to the entire wait-ing room, 'And every one of them, they gave me three months to live!' Among my patients, Irma is one such example. However, this actually happens infrequently in any one doctor's career. The main reason doctors avoid discussing a prognosis is because they don't know how. Most of us have never been shown how and have never seen somebody do it in real life. Unbelievable as it may seem, we learn to answer this most fundamental of questions by stumbling through grounds rich with our own trial and error, missed opportunities and inaccurate guesses. During training there is the obligatory lecture or two on delivering bad news, but it falls far short of replicating either the patient's or the doctor's dread when the real situation arises.

Sensing my reluctance, she says, 'It would be unfair for my children to not even have an idea.'

'Alana, if the cancer keeps growing at this rate, you probably have several weeks to a few months only.'

She draws in her breath sharply.

Mike, silent until now, speaks up. 'Are you sure? I think we should get a second opinion.'

My heart sinks. His tone is laden with recrimination and I fear that my doubts have succeeded in contaminating his initial confidence in me. When a patient asks to seek a second opinion, it can be hard not to treat the gesture as a personal affront. But one only has to consider what is at stake – life itself – before acknowledging its justification. I find my initial reaction replaced by relief. Perhaps another oncologist will be less pessimistic and lend her the hope that I have just vaccumed from her heart.

'Mike, I think getting a second opinion may be a good idea for you both. I am happy to arrange it.'

But Alana steps in. 'No, I don't need a second opinion because I think you are right. I have felt terrible all along and I'm actually relieved that there is a reason for it. I found it hard when everyone was doing their best to help me and nothing seemed to work – at least I know I wasn't making it up.'

'If you change your mind, I would be happy to do so anyway.'

I am again impressed by her calm as she addresses questions that she has obviously thought about deeply before today. It is also clear that the latest news has prompted her to resume control of her situation, whereas she was previously happy for me to make decisions on her behalf. She reminds me of this when she asks if she can step outside for a few minutes to talk to her husband in private. When they return, she says, 'I hope you don't think me foolish, but I have decided not to have any more treatment. It might have a chance of working, but I don't want to feel any worse and I really want to take my children on a holiday while I am still able to. I know that this may be our last time together and I feel as if they need something good to remember this whole thing by.'

My throat constricts at the sincerity, poise and dignity with which she says this, neither indulging in nor inviting pity. I am reminded again of the random opportunities I am provided to witness human sacrifice and resilience at its finest. When I look sideways at her husband, he seems conflicted and sad. His eyes are red and his grip on her hand has not once relaxed. 'How do you feel about this?' sounds so trivial that instead I simply reach for her outstretched hand. 'I think what you are doing is admirable.'

Alana and her family enjoy a trouble-free holiday for two weeks. She has my number but doesn't call me. As I watch other patients grapple with similar momentous decisions and vacillate between a selection of dismal options, my regard grows for her decisiveness.

'We had a great time!' she enthuses on her return.

'What did you do?' I ask curiously. She has grown too weak to enjoy her favourite pastime of hiking. She has lost her famous zeal for eating at restaurants and she is unable to stay awake for a movie.

'Mostly we sat around and talked. We talked about our lives, tried to make sense of our family's destiny and think of ways in which each of the kids could remember the good things we have done together. We also took pictures and made a video.' She stops for a moment before carrying on. 'I can tell you this because you are a mother too. I was worried about what to say to the children. Do I pretend I am okay? Do I invite their questions or discourage them? Would our talks be too much for them to bear? You know, when you are diagnosed with cancer, no one warns you that some of the most burdensome and painful times are not going through treatment but when you counsel your children. Teaching your children how to come to terms with your death is not how you ever imagine a family holiday, but all three of them said they felt much better for our talks.'

I think of my last holiday with my children at the beach. We built sandcastles, caught waves and watched in awe as the sun went down in a gloriously painted sky. The most difficult question we dealt with was which flavour of ice cream to have next.

'I know things are getting worse, my breathing especially. But I don't need to tell you that. You are the doctor . . .'

'I can learn much from you as a mother,' I respond.

She beams at the compliment. 'That's the nicest thing any doctor has ever said to me!' she exclaims, her face blazing with pride.

It was the last time I heard her speak. Barely two weeks later, she is rushed to hospital on a Friday evening. An urgent scan reveals her lungs to be drowning in cancer and she also has pneumonia. Treatment is begun with antibiotics, oxygen and fluids. When I walk into her room on Saturday morning, I don't recognise the person sitting up in bed, propped up and supported by a large number of pillows. Her weight has simply fallen away. Sweat drains off her face and drips into the oxygen mask that hangs limply from her chin as she wipes her face. Her sparse, wet hair is plastered against her skull. The enviable self-assurance she exuded just two weeks ago is gone, replaced by fear that I can smell. I am shocked at her transformation.

'She has lost her voice,' Mike says. 'She just can't talk. They said that the cancer has invaded an important nerve, that's why.'

'That's right,' I say gently, as I make my way to examine Alana.

'Hello, Alana.' She sits quietly, despondently. Mike helps me support her weight as I listen to the uncanny rattling of her chest. Her pulse feels weak. She is dying.

The young intern accompanying me says, 'She has had diarrhoea and there is a question about whether it's something serious. We are waiting to collect more blood and stool samples but they are proving hard to get. We might get the anaesthetist to put in a drip.' He looks satisfied at his precise summary of the situation. I groan silently.

'Alana, you have pneumonia. We are treating you with powerful antibiotics. Are you comfortable?'

She avoids eye contact and sinks exhaustedly into the narrow bed. I let go of her hand. I look at Mike, who has nothing to add.

The rest of the weekend ward round pressing on me, I move towards the exit. As we make for the next patient, the intern speaks again. 'Would you believe it, she wanted to be discharged home today, and I said no way, she was too sick to go anywhere for a while!'

I stop in my tracks. 'She asked to go home?'

'Asked? She can't talk but she sure knows how to get mad. Some people just can't figure out what's best for them.'

I retrace my steps. Alone and turned to one side, Alana is

looking out of the window at the beautiful afternoon of a waning winter. I walk around her bed so I can face her. I kneel on the floor beside her.

'Alana, I hear you asked to go home.'

She opens her mouth to speak but realises she can't. She reaches out for a whiteboard and pen on the side table. 'Send me home!' she scribbles, then holds the whiteboard up for me.

'As soon as you improve.'

'This won't get better,' she writes, fixing me with a stare. She knows that I know she is right.

'Antibiotics can treat the infection, make you less breathless. It's worth a try.'

She circles her first statement. 'Send me home.' There is a maniacal expression in her eyes.

I desperately look around for Mike to help my case. 'Alana, stay for the weekend at least. You might feel a lot better.'

She cannot argue with me for she has neither the voice nor the strength. But her eyes are brimming with despair. I have never seen her look so troubled before.

'Why do you want to go home today?'

She looks at me and shakes her head with disappointment. Grabbing a corner of her bed sheet, she clears the whiteboard before writing again. 'Die at home, with kids.'

So she too knows the end is near. I should have expected her to make her own decisions to the last.

'Alana, you are so sick I don't see how we can get you home. You will need oxygen, antibiotics . . . I don't think you should go yet.'

'Be with kids. Don't abandon me now.'

She is done with the whiteboard. She throws it on the floor and covers her face. I am rattled, deeply uncomfortable and conflicted.

But I also vividly remember the sense of unfinished business that hung over me for a long time when a patient with liver metastases never made it home, spending each precious day in the hope of an unachievable miracle. That experience forever changed my way of thinking about which hospital admissions to consider necessary.

Outside her room, I tell the intern, 'Okay, let us get her home.'

He stares at me. 'We can't do that!'

'You heard her.'

Sensing my hesitation, he feels emboldened. 'We have a duty of care to her.'

I look at his young, pained expression, probably trying to recollect what he ought to do when he so clearly disagrees with his boss. I could simply exert my rank but I want to and, in fact, need to have this argument with someone who can talk back to me.

'So what would you say is our duty of care to her?'

'To treat what we can and ease her suffering.'

'And if we can't do either?'

'To tell ourselves that at least we tried.'

Despite my irritation, I am impressed with the intern's stance. I tell myself that it is not fair to exclude this as a teaching moment. We go back to Alana's bedside. She hasn't moved. Her husband has returned and stands at the head of her bed. I take a deep breath.

'Alana, I know how devoted you are to your children and how desperate you are to be home with them. If we keep you in, there is a small chance that you will improve. But if I let you go, you will die.'

She looks up at me and nods. She removes her oxygen mask and looks me in the eye. I pick up her fallen whiteboard and give it to her. She writes without taking her eyes off me.

'We talked about this on our holiday.' Then she draws another circle around 'Send me home.'

'Alana, you are going home.'

Her defeated expression changes in a split second. Tears fall from her eyes as her hand grasps Mike's. 'Thank you,' she mouths.

The intern watches the scene in total silence, awed by what he has seen unfold. He follows me outside.

'Any other questions?'

'No.'

She is the one of the quickest weekend discharges I have ever seen. No sooner have we told the nurses than Mike's paramedic friends bring around an ambulance to transport them home. Someone finds a spare cylinder of oxygen that will be sufficient for the weekend. We give her an extra shot of antibiotics and enough pain relief to ease the journey back. As she is loaded onto the stretcher, she looks content despite her laboured breathing and uncomfortable posture. She even manages to raise her right hand to wave at us. As I watch the ambulance recede from the hospital, I finally feel my job is done.

She dies on Sunday, twenty-four hours after getting home. She was surrounded by her three children and conscious until the last few hours when she drifted off into a final sleep. I express my regret to Mike that I could not do any more to help her.

'She was happy,' Mike said. 'She was afraid that she would be trapped in hospital and pleaded with me not to take her there. When they said she couldn't go home, I felt I would carry the guilt all my life. She always knew she was dying and she had said to me she wanted her final memory to be of our home, where we have lived ever since we got married. Our children were born there and it was the place where she found the most happiness.'

Several weeks later, I receive a note in the mail. It is from Mike. He has sent me a copy of a painting that their young daughter did at school. The painting depicts her mother lying in bed. She is thin and looks small but is smiling. Around her are gathered three stick figures, depicting her children. At the end of the bed is her father, carrying a glass of water. He is smiling too. The picture is titled simply, 'The day my Mummy came home'.

10

◇

We will figure it out

I keep wishing I had never met her. On the day, I happen to be on the medical ward to find a file when a colleague pulls me aside. 'Will you have a look at this poor woman? She has been here for a month but I don't think oncology has seen her yet.'

With time on my hands, I agree, mainly to rectify the situation of a delayed consult. I soon discover why.

Already, her file is as thick as that of someone who has spent several months in hospital. She is seventy-four years old, a visitor from Bangladesh, here to see her six children. Months into her visit, she developed acute and progressive difficulty swallowing, until she came to hospital complaining of breathlessness. Tests revealed a cancer in her rib eroding through into the lung, creating an abscess. There is concern that the abscess might also harbour tuberculosis. The complicated abscess has needed repeated draining and the insertion of a tube. So far, she has largely been in the hands of the surgeon, whose preoccupation it has been to ensure that her infected lung heals. But the insulted lung has resisted sterilisation. Unless the infection is cured, there can be no talk of chemotherapy, so the oncology consult has rightly been deferred week after week.

Locating her isolation bay on the ward, I knock and enter. A pleasant-looking young woman, the patient's daughter, greets me, followed by a man who identifies himself as her brother. The elderly man who rises next must be the patient's husband. The patient herself is lying in bed, a thin woman with clear skin and a narrow but expressive face. Her hair is tied back in a knot. The chest tube pokes through the side of the bed, draining into a bag. Her expression changes from disinterest to curiosity when I mention my Indian name.

'My parents don't understand English. My name is Amit,' her son offers.

I ask her son whether he is abreast of her situation. He nods shyly, not the type to ask questions.

'My job later will be to talk about cancer treatment but we have to wait till the damaged lung has healed.' I calculate that this may take weeks, even months.

She did not take out travel insurance and every day in the hospital is expensive, what with the cost of the repeated operations, specialised equipment and medication. At first glance, this looks to be a family of modest means, but I could be wrong. I leave the room after a few minutes, my involvement still premature. Over the next several weeks, I drop in on her occasionally, each time only to discover that her progress has been marginal. I wonder how long the family can keep pace with the mounting bills. One day I bring up the issue with her son.

'What do you plan to do once she is out of hospital?'

'I think we will send her back home to Bangladesh. Cancer treatment here would be too expensive.'

I relax. A few weeks later, I receive a call from the patient's treating physician. 'The lung is on the mend and we are discharging her. She needs to be seen by so many different specialities that it would be nice if you could coordinate her care while she remains in the country.'

'Sure.' This is how I came to inherit Mrs Bala, thinking it would be a straightforward task to see that she travelled to Bangladesh with the necessary paperwork outlining her treatment to date.

The first time I see them in my clinic is also the first time in two months that I have seen her out of bed. Her average height is accentuated by her thin build. She is bent forward a little, as if coaxing her body out of pain. She wears a plain but clean sari and her black hair is neatly swept back. Although she does not say a word, her entire demeanour is pleasant, non-threatening and, in some way, soothing. She could be anyone's mother, I think, including my own. I take her hand and help her sit down in a chair next to her husband. Amit tells me that the surgeon was happy with her progress although warned that she was not yet out of the woods and needed to be on antibiotics.

'They said you would tell us what to do about the cancer,' he says.

I ask if she is going to Bangladesh to have treatment.

'No, she is too weak to fly, and my parents have no supports there. She is staying with us for the time being.'

That sounds fine, I think, but how will they afford cancer treatment? The generous health system is funded by the government for those who are fortunate enough to be residents, but visitors are liable for prohibitive bills.

It seems cruel to begin the discussion of treatment with its likely inaffordability, but equally so to promise it without explaining the terms. Yet, it's not my job, I reason. It's not my job to mete out treatment according to ability to pay. The first of many debates to come enters my head. How should a discussion with a patient be affected by their ability to pay, for the consultation or the treatment? As new, so-called 'blockbuster' drugs enter the market, it is becoming every physician's dilemma to deal with the consequences. Many of these drugs cost thousands, even hundreds of thousands of dollars, often for a gain in longevity of weeks. Patients and their families can become bankrupt in the process of funding the latest miracle drug, tempted by the thought that they may be the one case in a million to achieve a long-lasting remission or a cure. Most often, though, the only tangible result seems to be a mountain of debt.

The chemotherapy that Mrs Bala needs consists of generic drugs that cost relatively little, but it is the cost of administering them, and the medical and nursing support required, that will prove expensive. Scans done in hospital show that Mrs Bala's cancer is localised. Were it not for the perforation into the lung, it may even have been curable. Now, the situation is not so straightforward, even from a strictly medical viewpoint. I have a dull feeling that I already know her fate.

'There are a few different ways in which we could try to treat the cancer, but a lot depends on how the lung heals.'

'The doctors are really happy with it.'

'That's good! Bear with me while I talk to a radiation doctor.'

I hunt out the kindest of the radiation oncologists to talk about my dilemma. In my previous dealings, I have always found him to be sensible and sensitive.

'I guess it comes down to two questions,' I end. 'One, would you give her radiotherapy? Two, could you do it free of charge?'

He cups his chin in his hands and thinks for a while, staring and sighing at the scans. And then he finally says, 'I am glad I don't have to deal with the second question because I don't think anyone would risk giving her radiotherapy.'

My heart sinks.

'The fistula into her lung is still healing. Radiotherapy risks reopening the passage. I would be seriously concerned that she would have a few days of radiotherapy, which would not affect the cancer, but be sufficient to result in life-threatening sepsis.'

'Is there anyone else who could do something different?' I plead. 'Do you want to discuss her case with your colleagues?'

He looks at me sympathetically.

'I hate this too. But we come across a handful of such cases, and every time we have decided against radiation because the benefits just aren't there and the risk is fatal.'

'I knew it didn't look good,' I say dejectedly.

'I am sorry. This is terrible, especially for something that could have been potentially curable.'

On the way back to my office, I run into another oncologist and ask how he would treat Mrs Bala. He says without hesitation that he would steer well away from chemotherapy too. 'A single drop in her cell counts and she could be in deep trouble.' In saying this, he mirrors my own views.

I return to my room where the family looks up expectantly. How does a doctor convey the news that no one is willing to treat a patient?

I start. 'We feel that the risk of treatment is too high and could reactivate the lung abscess.' It is obvious as they wait for more that they have not made the required leap of logic.

'So the abscess needs more treatment.'

'Yes,' I respond gently. 'But we cannot start treating the cancer yet. Perhaps she will be a lot better in a month's time and we can revisit the issue.' I try to be encouraging but I am sure that we will be having the same conversation again.

'So what are you going to do about the cancer?'

'Just keep an eye on it.'

The more I use this euphemism for a variety of situations, the more rankled I feel by its hollow promise.

'But how is that possible?'

'We watch out for any symptoms, such as pain or weight loss, or growing fatigue.'

'And then what?'

'We see what we can do.'

The family's lack of conviction competes in intensity with my own. I know that although she is stable now, these symptoms will eventually appear. And there will be no treatment then as there is none now because the first principle every doctor will wish to follow is 'First, do no harm'. There may be help around the edges, something for her nausea, something for her pain, but not their ultimate cause. But none of this truth seems as clear-cut to the patient or her family. It is confronting and painful to predict the future; today, I simply hang onto the hope that doctors have been known to be wrong even in their most certain predictions.

'Does your mother have any questions for me? Can you make sure she understands?'

There is unintelligible conversation in Bengali; even to my foreign ears, the few words exchanged seem inadequate to summarise all that I have said. I can only trust the family to do my bidding in good faith.

'Can we come back to see you, doctor?'

What does the hospital want them to do? Pay for each doctor's visit? What does the hospital want me to do? Stop dispensing at my will the time it pays me for?

'Sure you can.'

'Do we have to pay?'

'You don't have to pay me personally.'

I can find no other polite way of warning them that somewhere within the bowels of bureaucracy, there may be somebody whose job it is to reprise every interaction they have with me.

'Thank you.'

I see them every two weeks because this is the longest the family can go without reassurance. Mrs Bala's cancer turns out to be highly aggressive, resulting in progressive weight loss. She has a feeding tube inserted through her nose but the tube is too thin to allow meaningful feeding. She begins to lose condition. Her dietitian sends me a note painstakingly detailing her concerns if the weight loss continues unchecked. But what touches me is that the young dietitian has made private arrangements to see Mrs Bala and stays in frequent touch on the phone with them so they don't incur a charge. She has used her connections to obtain them cheaper supplements and for someone overworked and under-resourced, she has gone out of her way to invest in one patient. I have never met her but I realise that she is one of the many unheralded people who form the backbone of the work that doctors and nurses receive predominant credit for.

'You have a wonderful dietitian,' I say, wondering whether they are aware of how extraordinary the service is that she is providing them.

They nod.

I don't mention to them the dietitian's frustration at the inadequacy of Mrs Bala's feeding tube, evident when she writes in her note, 'I don't mean to tell you what to do but have you considered a PEG?'

A PEG is also a feeding device, directly inserted into the stomach, making nutrition easier. But its risks can be potentially more serious too. By this time, the first bill of tens of thousands of dollars has arrived and I feel loath to even mention another expense.

Mrs Bala battles on, with sporadic visits to other doctors who slowly wind up their peripheral involvement. The next time I see her, her head is bowed and her frame has grown even more gaunt. She acknowledges me with dull eyes and allows me to examine her without the slightest resistance or interest. She behaves and must feel like a mannequin.

'I can't find anything obvious, like an infection, and we know that the tests for TB were negative,' I say. 'But that is not to say that you feel well,' I hurriedly add. There is nothing that irritates patients more than being told there is nothing wrong with them when they feel they will never rise from their bed again.

Everyone nods. No one translates. It is as if they expected nothing more from me.

Having now seen her many times, a familiar sense of frustration rises within me as I realise that I have no idea what she feels, wants or fears. She is seated before me but she is incalculably distant. The lack of a common language between us not only makes any conversation impossible but also dilutes the empathy that I experience for her. There is nothing like a patient saying, 'I feel terrible and I want you to help me' to bring suffering home. But filtered through the patina of the whimsical tongue of relatives, any sentiment, however powerful, is lost in translation. Even the most competent, professional interpreter relays only what the patient explicitly states; nothing can capture the nuanced exchange between a doctor and patient, which may be framed by words but relies heavily on the buttress of body language, meaningful silence and the mutual understanding of cues. I try to shake off the feeling that I am treating a theoretical patient, but I know that my conversation could plumb greater depths if we could communicate directly.

'Is there anything your mother wants to know?' I ask Amit.

'Um . . . not really.'

'That can't be right!' I want to retort. 'She is slowly wasting away from an untreated cancer and you are telling me that she is not curious. Either you are holding back information or she is protecting you from her concerns and fears!'

'People in your mother's situation can have a number of questions about the present and future,' I persist.

'I think she is pretty accepting.'

I can only hope that his assessment of his mother's Zen-like attitude is accurate. But it doesn't take too much to suspect that she is troubled. Is she troubled by her current symptoms or the uncertain future? How will I find out?

The next time, all her children attend the consultation, usually a sign of escalating anxiety. They come straight to the point.

'People tell us that we should send our mother back to Bangladesh.'

Their mother is a mere shadow of herself, if this were possible with the small reserve she started out with. She braces her chest with both hands when she coughs. Her tears drop at the mere effort of this exercise. Suddenly I am filled with trepidation for her.

'People say that she could get better care there.'

This dispassionate statement is like a punch in the gut, the most direct insinuation there can be that my care is lacking. A mixture of indignation and bitterness washes over me and my immediate instinct is to leap to my own defence and that of my unstinting colleagues.

I rein in my tongue. I have learnt over the years that the nebulous 'they' is a synonym patients and families use for 'I' and 'we'. 'They think I should give up treatment' means 'I can't bear the thought of more chemotherapy'. 'They say my morphine could go up' hints at worsening pain and the need for the doctor to acknowledge it. It can be arduous to read between the lines but I try.

'What do you think?'

'We just want what is best for our mother.'

I suddenly feel as if I am counsel for the defence. How did I get here?

'Maybe there would be a regular doctor there . . .' Her daughter leaves the thought hanging in the air.

A more regular doctor than one who allocates a free long consultation every fortnight? I have been her advocate through the months and have spent countless hours organising her care. The family has my details on speed dial and makes ready use of them. It would require a superhuman effort not to feel slighted. But I remind myself that professionalism is easy with a patient who likes you and values your opinion. In some ways, the true test is presented by the likes of Mrs Bala and her family.

'Tell me what I can do to help.'

'We don't mind your care but it's just other people who think differently.'

I take a deep breath. 'If you want to take her back, I will do everything possible to help you.'

'Don't take her home!' my mind screams. 'Her case is too complex and she is too sick for another doctor to pick up the pieces now. Just let her be.'

'Do you think she could receive better treatment there?'

I, like many others, dislike answering this question. Every doctor feels the need to initiate independent investigations to arrive at an independent conclusion. How many new tests will Mrs Bala have to endure again and for what purpose? Will they wither away her fragile reserve? What if someone, not comprehending the true complexity of her condition, felt game enough to treat her and caused the disastrous complications that we have feared? It would be far too late for the family to regret the move then.

'What would you do?' someone prompts.

Instead of answering their question, I ask them one in return: 'Who would go back with your mother?'

'Just our father.'

'Does he think he could manage to care for her?'

'No, he is afraid he will be all alone.'

For a fleeting minute, Mrs Bala's children feel like my siblings; I feel desperate to avert them from self-inflicted harm.

'You need to be prepared that if she returns, you will not see her again.'

'Oh.'

There is a yawning silence in the room. I feel sorry for them if they are only just realising this truth. Why is it that the most self-evident statements draw the biggest surprise?

Finally, the truth emerges, something that should have been evident to me.

'I guess we are worried how much more this could cost us.' Amit says this with obvious distaste and discomfort. His siblings look down.

'Of course.' I can find no other words.

From the way she looks, I expect to see her in hospital again. They look at me mutely. They are proud migrants, used to standing on their feet and solving their own problems. But this one seems genuinely beyond them. I don't want to know what work they do because it will only compound our mutual unease. On the odd occasion when I have called her son, he has answered his phone surreptitiously, saying he is not allowed to talk on the job.

'Can you pay your current bill?' This seems a question no less intrusive.

'It's going to be hard.' I note that it's not a flat negative.

They are determined not to ask for help. I sense a whiff of hostility but I can't imagine why this could be. Are they blaming me for advising she stay where she is? Do they hold me responsible that her disease cannot be treated? I know that I need to do something for her sake, to release her of the duty she must feel towards her children facing this unprecedented situation. What mother would not groan at becoming a burden to her children?

'I will speak to someone, don't pay the bill just yet.'

Again, the same detachment.

Tracking 'someone' down is harder than I realised. It takes numerous phone calls and enquiries to find the right person. It takes days to have the call returned. The officer is polite but noncommittal. Upon hearing my rendering of Mrs Bala's predicament, he responds that at any one time he is presented with a handful of such cases, each vying for extra compassion.

'You have to realise we can't simply keep forgiving these large debts. People choose not to take out insurance but when they fall sick, they cost a lot of money and someone has to take on the cost. You will understand that cancer patients are particularly expensive to the system.' He goes on to tell me about the number of visitors who default on their bills and the arduous task of weighing up whether to pursue them. He refers to the health care systems of other nations, including Mrs Bala's home, where one would not get past the door without payment. And he casually mentions the moral difficulty in elevating one terrible illness over another.

'And before you say it, doctor,' he says with a laugh, but only half-jokingly, 'I have heard "But my patient has cancer" four times this week.'

The rest of my plea evaporates. 'See what you can do. Thank you for listening.'

'Send in a form and I will have a look.'

The conversation deflates me but his argument makes sense. It is his role to safekeep the finances of an entire health care system, so that mounting debts don't bring all our functions to a halt. His is a job beyond my comprehension. My task is to serve the individual patient, preferably in the most cost-efficient manner so as to consider overall societal good, but I am well aware that from time to time, I have the luxury of disregarding the second clause.

I reflect that what is good for Mrs Bala is not good for the hospital. It would have been ideal if she had gone back home at diagnosis, like many visitors opt to. But what Mrs Bala needs at this late stage is the care and compassion of her family, who have built their lives here. She will need medical intervention from time to time but the most important aspect of her care is now human contact. How to draw the attention and compassion of a bureaucracy that serves millions to the needs of one individual? I say the patient is the first of her kind I have seen in many years; the hospital says it copes with a few of them every week.

It takes me another week to find out that there is no official form to plead for special financial dispensation for patients. 'You will just have to write a convincing letter,' the social worker says sympathetically.

The letter takes longer than I would have thought. My words must argue for consideration and generosity of spirit but they must also contain truth – about her likelihood of needing more medical help and the family's risk of defaulting on payment. The hospital has already indicated that it would be more willing to consider debt reduction if there were an end point to the medical interventions, but I feel strongly that Mrs Bala's interests would be best served by staying on. I feel saddened by the need to argue her case but try not to become so enveloped in the fog of idealism that I lose objectivity. I feel better when the letter is sent.

She develops a hacking cough and pain, and needs morphine. My boss generously agrees for our department's discretionary funds to assume the major cost of her expensive painkillers. Her lack of adequate feeding continues to be a thorny issue for the family.

Tired of falsely reassuring them, I contact the PEG team.

The junior doctor laughs at me. 'We would never put a PEG into someone like her.' Piqued at her insouciance, I write a letter to the specialist, who surprises me by acceding to my request. The PEG tube is successfully placed; everyone is relieved. But I am seared by the words of the nurse: 'These patients have a high mortality rate. She was a borderline case but we gave her the benefit of the doubt because you said so.'

To my growing fear, being fed larger amounts through the PEG tube does not make an appreciable difference to Mrs Bala's well-being. I wish again that she would make an attempt to talk to me or answer my questions with more than a monosyllable, but she seems to have given up hope.

'Have you heard about the bill yet?' I enquire. 'I sent the letter some time ago.'

'Finance has been in touch. They were considering your letter but they did say not to worry, that they would help us.'

'Did they say what sort of help?'

'I think they said we wouldn't have to pay anything.'

Despite the prompting it required and the complacency with which this news is relayed, I feel joyful. I had little expectation of finance coming up with a complete solution to my problem, which they had made clear was far from unique. I feel grateful to the officer and proud of the institution which has found it within its heart to make this gesture.

'I am very glad. That's great news!'

Mrs Bala raises her hand gratefully, showing that she has gleaned the substance of the conversation. Her son stays silent. I resolve to keep feeling good about the fact that my hospital has just swallowed tens of thousands of dollars of her debt.

Driving home that evening, I can't help wondering why

Mrs Bala's family practises such obvious reserve in the face of my redoubled efforts to help her. How can they possibly not appreciate the time and energy that I spend on her case while queues of patients wait patiently outside? Is a simple thank you from time to time too much to ask? I know that this is not why I do the work I do, but I can't help feeling unappreciated after many tough rounds of negotiations with so many people for Mrs Bala's sake. The family is not rude or argumentative, but I am convinced that nothing short of a revised diagnosis will please them. I have a sinking feeling that the more I try to help, the higher they will raise the bar. All my life, I have practised jumping bars, for this is how one becomes a doctor. But even I am growing weary of this moving bar.

Despite the attitude of her family, Mrs Bala's case gets under my skin for a different reason. Having lived an itinerant life myself, the story of an old lady stuck with an untreatable cancer in a foreign land affects me deeply and I find myself dwelling on her misfortune. Without realising it, I become irritable. After dealing with the intense emotion and hard work of looking after a non-communicative but desperately needy patient, I cannot find a tolerant ear for a friend who complains of having her second cold this month or my husband, who cannot locate our daughter's dummy.

'Everything else seems so insignificant,' I complain loudly into the air.

My son appeals to me in a very reasonable tone: 'But, Mama, just find the dummy!'

His unarguable claim is a timely reminder that seemingly superhuman efforts at work do not absolve one from finding elusive objects at home. Some days the transition from doctor to mother feels like a rapid and turbulent mid-air descent, but one that is important to keep me grounded. One of the best things I learnt from an old professor is that no one is indispensable. He was scheduled for serious surgery and I asked how he was preparing to relinquish control of his vast practice. 'My patients will manage just fine. It is whether I will manage without their needing me.' I think of his words now.

I refer Mrs Bala to palliative care. The nurse says it won't be straightforward. 'Does she have a family doctor?' he asks.

'No. I am her doctor.'

'She will need someone to certify her when she dies, unless you want to travel to wherever she lives.'

I groan. The complications just keep coming.

'Leave it with me.'

Later that day, I receive a call in the middle of a clinic. It is Amit, clearly panicking.

'My mother can't breathe. I will put her next to the phone. Can you hear her?' A faint shrieking and at times piercing sound comes over the line – Mrs Bala sounds as if she is choking. 'She has been like this the whole night.'

Asking my patient to step outside, I think of summoning an ambulance to Mrs Bala's aid, but mindful of the cost, I change my mind and call the hospice.

'Get them to bring her here straight away. We will save our last bed.'

Immensely grateful at being able to expedite her care, I tell Amit to rush her to the hospice.

The next call I receive is from a nurse: 'I thought you would like to know that Mrs Bala died within minutes of arriving here. We gave her a little bit of morphine but she died before we could start anything else.'

I feel stunned, part of a horror movie. My first instinct is to reach for Amit's phone number.

'Is her family still there?' I ask the nurse.

'Yes. They are all with her.'

'Thank you for letting me know.'

'That's okay. It sounded like you did a lot.'

Having located Amit's number, I dial it but hang up before it is answered. No, the family needs time to come to terms with this devastating and unexpected end. I wait all day for him to call. The family makes no attempt to reach me. My mind burns with questions about the days leading up to her death. Why the calamitous decline? Could it have been prevented? Was she in pain? Did no one recognise her breathing to be abnormal or simply terrifying? And like all the other times, why didn't anyone call me sooner? Was it just a miscalculation or had they lost faith in me by then?

For many successive days, I toy with the idea of calling the family, a gesture that comes naturally when my patients die. But there was something in their conduct that repeatedly turns me away from making the call. I can't shake the feeling that they hold me responsible in some way for her entire journey with cancer, and I don't want to inflame the situation. Perhaps they are waiting for my call, I tell myself. Perhaps they respect how busy I am or feel that I have moved on. But they have never before hesitated to call me – on weekends, public holidays and even Sunday mornings, knowing that I would always meet their needs. The days turn into weeks and into months. Like one jilted in love, I manufacture excuses while waiting for a call that will never come. It feels ridiculous and immature.

Oncology is a fragile business, overtly so for patients, but no less for the doctors who devote themselves to caring for these patients when they are at their rawest and most vulnerable. The moment the oncologist drops the bombshell of a cancer diagnosis and watches the lightning spread of fear, and the time when all therapies are exhausted and there is only comfort care to recommend to disbelieving ears – these are merely the sobering bookends. But in between lie the countless other occasions that are no less distressing. Occasions on which the promise of chemotherapy remains only that; when the most thorough tests do not pick up the advancing claw of cancer; when no one could have predicted the intensity of vomiting or the depth of fatigue. Or the times when the spouse-turned-carer suddenly announces he is fleeing the marriage; when the estranged child refuses to reconcile; when a loan is needed to cover the cost of morphine.

Unlike a family doctor, no one *needs* an oncologist. One is sent to an oncologist when the situation prescribes it, but the relationship by its very nature soon turns into one of privileged intimacy. How can it be anything less when one meets a stranger confronted by a life-threatening diagnosis and within a few encounters becomes privy to his or her deepest thoughts on the matter of illness, destiny, religion, family and death? The ties that bind oncologist and patient can be warm and gratifying, a just reward for choosing to take on this demanding role that never ends at sunset.

It is important to breathe in the anguish of patients, and hurt enough to be meaningfully and compassionately involved in their care, but if I allow myself to become too entangled in the details of every patient's struggle, every Mrs Bala will seem like my mother and every patient's death will be a personal failure set to challenge my choices and my convictions. Treading the thin line between too little engagement and too much, especially at a time when doctors are increasingly believed to err on the side of the former, is hard and dangerous. One raises the unhappy spectre of dissatisfied patients and family, the other the occasional but real disappointment of going unthanked and unacknowledged. Weighing up these possibilities, recognising the inherent challenges of treating the whole patient and not just the disease, and constantly steering towards doing what is right, not just expedient, is an exercise in loneliness. This loneliness is as intensely personal as it must be common, for what I deal with is a small fraction of the load carried by the busiest among us. But the task of dealing with desperately ill patients, lending them minute parcels of hope to be snatched away without notice, watching them die premature deaths while you and your children thrive, is a heavy and private cross to bear. It is the silent price of being an oncologist.

Carrying the matter of Mrs Bala's family like a wound that is insolently slow to heal, I talk to my close friend. He is a family doctor, loved and trusted by his patients, and endowed with many more years of experience and wisdom than me. We recall wading through weeks of our training dedicated to being mindful of our patients. We learnt about fostering and honouring the doctor-patient relationship but also the avenues disaffected patients could pursue, ranging from complaining to the hospital, the ombudsman, the police, the coroner, or the medical registration board. We recall being ourselves subjected to these anxieties, thankfully only rarely and ultimately without substance, but not before they had created a period of total havoc in our lives. But we never learnt anything about coping with that other aspect of a long career – patients and relatives who are abusive, unreasonable or, for other reasons, just disappointing. They are thankfully not common but any doctor who has come across one knows the deep impact their behaviour leaves. Without having any ready answers, he talks about his similar experiences and I feel better for knowing them.

Closure on Mrs Bala will never come. Mainly, my mind wanders back to the most basic questions that go to the core of why I chose to become an oncologist. They all have to do with providing comfort. Was the morphine I prescribed enough? Did they run out of the small bottle because that's all I could procure for them on the day? Why did they wait so late before they called me? Who, if anyone, talked them through the possibility of her imminent death? And after all the efforts, did they finally end up with their debt forgiven?

I have decided never to call them. They have clearly decided the same. I concede that sometimes we all need to insulate ourselves from more hurt, and that, as in real life, the practice of medicine serves up rejections that are hard to swallow.

Everyone needs to define a way of reconciling to these inevitable bumps. Some, like my friend, seek consolation in the keys of an old, loved piano. Others paint, pray, run or meditate. I seek silent refuge in my writing, sometimes losing myself happily to the wonder of how arrangements of a mere twenty-six letters can erase dejection and restore clarity of thought. I also find consolation in a myriad other forms – a stable family, the unbridled happiness of my young children, my own good health, and the company of surviving patients whose thanks should go to the intrinsic behaviour of their cancer rather than the 'miraculous' powers wielded by their oncologist.

The week after Mrs Bala's death, I meet a brand new patient. She is eighty, from a Pacific island. Her visitor's visa expires this week and when she was having it renewed, she fainted in the queue. She is bleeding from an advanced rectal cancer and can't even sit comfortably. She only speaks an island dialect.

Her daughter pleads tearfully, 'Doctor, I know she doesn't have long but please help me keep her in my house. She has no one back home.'

I take a deep breath, stifling the ache that threatens to rise again. As I look at the frail mother and her desperate daughter, everything about them screams hard work. I cannot imagine returning to the finance department with another plea so close on the heels of the first. But as I look at the elderly lady, sitting helplessly and appearing vulnerable, it seems petty to be consumed by my own misgivings. There is little place for self-pity in a career where a thousand more real tragedies vie for attention.

'Don't worry, we will figure it out. Let's start with some basic details.'

I I

◇

Why can't they all be like Peter?

It is a bitterly cold and uncomfortable winter night, the sort when the most natural thing to do is curl up on the floor and gaze dreamily at the leaping tongues of a cheerily lit fire. I am staying alone in a cosy rented apartment in a new city, where I have come to complete the final six months of my specialist oncology training.

After completing their local training, it is popular for doctors to spend a stint of time abroad, gaining a different perspective in their field. I have recently won a Fulbright Award to complete a fellowship at the University of Chicago, which has one of the oldest and most prestigious medical ethics programs in the world. Everything I have heard so far, as well as my interview with the medical faculty, has lit up my imagination. Twelve months immersed in a program that deals with real-life communication and ethical dilemmas in medicine, many of them involving cancer patients and their end of life care, seems an ideal way to round off my training as an oncologist. My husband has already left for Chicago, furthering his medical degree with a business one. Some of my closest friends and family live in the United States, where I spent my teenage years and completed high school. There are many reasons to be excited about the upcoming year.

The shrill ring of the phone breaks into my thoughts; I groan as I get up to answer it. A seventy-year-old patient has suddenly taken a turn for the worse.

'What's the matter?' I ask the intern.

'He is confused and looks unwell. It's hard to get much out of him as he can't speak clearly at the best of times.'

I give the intern some advice before reluctantly extinguishing the fire.

At the patient's bedside, I immediately see the reason for the intern's concern. The man is thrashing in bed, sweat dripping from his forehead as he gesticulates wildly at the staff. Gleaning a history from him is impossible and I set about trying to calm him down in order to examine him. Many possibilities go through my mind – he could be having a heart attack, stroke or internal bleeding. This is going to be a long night of phone calls to relatives, ordering tests and treating his problem. Instructing his nurse, I walk outside to the desk to sit down with his voluminous notes to create some order out of his presentation. As I start to wade through the paperwork, with one eye on the patient, a figure walks past me before turning back and approaching the desk.

'Hi! You are up late. Is everything okay?'

I recognise him as a surgeon at the hospital. I have seen him across the room at meetings but we have never exchanged a word in the few months that I have worked here. By all accounts, he is wildly popular. I am surprised he even knows who I am.

'I don't know yet. He is a transfer from surgery and he has suddenly become unwell.'

'Do you need a hand?'

'Oh no, I will figure it out.' I can't believe a senior surgeon would stop to volunteer help!

Just then the patient lets out a wild scream. I run into the room.

While I pummel the old man with questions he does not or cannot answer, I hear a soft voice behind me.

'Your patient is in urinary retention.'

I whip around to find the surgeon taking off his overcoat. He asks the nurse to prepare him a urinary catheter set to relieve the patient's bladder. I feel chastened by my failure to detect something so easy as I entertained a world of more complex diagnoses.

'I should have thought about it,' I say contritely. 'I will put in the catheter.'

'Are you sure? He probably has a large prostate.'

The sheer thought of traumatising a confused old man with repeated catheterisation tempts me to take up his offer, but the man screams again and I am convinced of the need for expediency over pride.

'I would be very grateful.'

As the nurse wheels in the catheter trolley, he strokes the patient's hand and talks to him in a calm voice. He continues to talk soothingly as he deftly guides the catheter into place. Urine gushes into the bag, accompanied by an instant expression of relief all around, not least on the face of the man, who looks exhausted from the effort of trying to tell us what was wrong. The clock in the room says one a.m.

I turn towards the surgeon. 'It is so good of you to help. Thank you.'

'It's good that he is resting again. He has already put up with a lot without needing additional worries.'

Far more used to taking orders from irate surgeons than accepting spontaneous gestures of goodwill, I am flabbergasted.

'Anyway, it's nice to meet you.'

As he leaves, a nurse sighs. 'Why can't they all be like Peter?'

My subsequent interactions with Peter are even more brief – at a morning presentation or a radiology meeting where we discuss operative patients. I find myself drawn to these meetings to hear Peter discuss his patients. His colleagues respect his technical proficiency and ask him for advice on difficult cases, but what I come to watch is his thoughtful dealing with the cases at hand. In a room full of doctors who know each other well and have worked together for many years, the conversations around patients are frank and sometimes brutally honest. One morning we are discussing a 47-year-old man who has recently been diagnosed with cancer of the pancreas. He is a prominent citizen, known for his philanthropy. Biting into a bagel, a surgeon says, 'Look at the scans. It's going to be a mess in there when I go in.'

Peter walks over to study the films. Standing next to him, even to my unpractised eye, the area looks mottled with cancer.

'Then maybe you shouldn't go in. It does look bad,' Peter says.

'But the guy is set on having an operation! He just doesn't get that he is going to be dead within a few months. His kid is graduating at the end of the year and another one is getting engaged and he wants to be around for all of the action!'

'All the more reason to talk him out of having a complicated operation,' Peter says mildly.

Silence descends on the room. A frank conversation about obstructive bureaucrats is one thing but talking a surgeon out of performing an operation is another. I steal a look at a colleague seated by me. She sips her coffee imperturbably while writing on her napkin, 'Go, Peter!'

The first surgeon speaks again, a subtle hint of ire in his tone: 'Peter, if I talk him out of having an operation, he will get someone else to do it.'

Aware of the delicate situation he has created, Peter neither backs down nor defends his position more aggressively. Instead he comments to no one in particular, 'I suppose the chap just needs to know that he could potentially spend whatever time he has left recovering from a major operation that does not cure him. I have had my share of those.'

I wait for the customary explosion of comments, but surprisingly no one has a contrary opinion. It is clear that even a gathering of famously independent-minded surgeons will take note of his words.

In the ensuing low-grade mumble, the first surgeon says, 'Look, I will have another chat to him, see whether he understands . . .'

Leaving the room with the consultant oncologist, I remark at the surgeon's turnaround that will spare an unknowing patient a complex and unnecessary operation.

The oncologist, who has known Peter for a long time, shakes her head. 'If I am ever sick, I would want him as my surgeon.'

A rewarding six months finally over, it is time for me to move on. At a morning meeting, Peter asks me about my plans. I casually mention to him that I am about to undertake a fellowship in medical ethics, feeling conscious that he may think I am wasting my time. But again, he surprises me with an appreciative discourse on the role of ethics in medicine.

'We take it for granted that as doctors we are conscientious. But the care of another sick human being brings up a lot of moral and ethical issues and we need doctors who can think deeply about them.' At a time in my career when I am still unsure of my professional bearings, I am tremendously reassured by his words.

Many months later a friend incidentally mentions in a phone call that Peter has been diagnosed with prostate cancer. He had been experiencing a nagging pain in his hip and although he was only in his forties, he became suspicious and had an X-ray. This is how he discovered that he had advanced prostate cancer. I am stunned by the news. I don't know how he dealt with the diagnosis but I am sure that it came as an enormous shock to a man who had led an exemplary life of work, exercise and overall well-being. I ask how he is doing.

'You wouldn't know it by looking at him,' she says before adding, 'but we are all very sad.'

I make up my mind to write to him to tell him how sorry I am to hear the news, but when I hang up the phone, I wonder whether he will even remember me and put off the letter. Inexplicably, a year goes by.

'He is doing incredibly well,' my friend tells me when I next ask about Peter. It seems too awkward to acknowledge the news now, I think, especially if he is so well. Coming from an oncologist, I fear it might be graceless to remind him of his condition. And he may yet have years to live if he is defying convention and doing so well.

I return to Australia with my husband after finishing our respective studies. When our first child is six months old, we return to Peter's city for a holiday. At the hospital where I used to work, and where he still does, I ask after him. There is a tinge of expectant sadness in the air, which makes me unable to decide whether to track him down. On one hand, he is one of the most striking people I have ever met, someone whose every action had a lesson within, someone who was looked upon as a real-life legend. On the other, I think, this is how I remember him from a few years ago. But has the diagnosis of cancer changed him? Will I still find him inspiring or has his inspiration been sapped by the sombreness of living a leased life?

Grappling with my indecision, I walk into the chemotherapy unit to greet erstwhile colleagues, where I find myself looking directly at Peter, snoozing in a reclining chair at the end of the room. It is late in the afternoon, when the usual babble of the chemotherapy unit has died down, replaced by a lull. Only a few patients remain. A bag of blood trickles slowly into an old lady's arm, an attempt to revitalise her from her lassitude, even if it is temporary. Another man laughs at a joke as his nurse detaches him from his intravenous pole. Peter sits well away and alone, in an annexe. Is it by design? I wonder. In a small hospital, it must be impossible to avoid running into his patients.

I know now that my decision has been made but I want to take my time in getting to Peter. Partly obscured by a desk while I chat to a nurse, I observe him. A bag of chemotherapy labelled with a coloured tag hangs from a pole above his chair. His eyes are closed and there is a peaceful expression on his face, which has not changed much from what I remember except it looks a little thinner. Two books are balanced on his outstretched legs, along with some writing paper and a broadsheet newspaper, folded in half. I smile. Peter has obviously not lost any of his drive to accomplish as much as possible at any given time. He suddenly opens his eyes and waves at me, his smile suggesting that he not only remembers me but is pleased to see me.

'How are you?' he asks before I can ask him the same question.

'Good, good!'

Perhaps to spare me the awkwardness, he offers, 'A little while after you left, I was diagnosed with metastatic prostate cancer. It's on the move again and I am having chemo.' He holds up his fingers, in cold gloves to protect the nails. 'Had much experience with this drug?'

'A little,' I say, not knowing what else to add. Many patients report brittle and discoloured nails from chemotherapy; the gloves are under study for their usefulness.

After briefly telling him about Chicago, and having started my career as a specialist oncologist since I last saw him, I ask, 'What do you do with yourself at home?' I am unable to imagine him at home and, apparently, so is he.

'Home?! I take a few days off around chemotherapy and then I am back operating again. I am busier than ever because I pack the same schedule into fewer days.'

I am taken aback by his revelation. In my clinic, I write out long-term medical and disability certificates for people far less sick than Peter. I can't believe that he continues to work full-time. Surely he does not need to; I am intrigued to know his reasons. As he talks, his eagerness to keep contributing to patient care, as well as teaching and mentoring trainee surgeons, is obvious. He treats his cancer as an inconvenience he needs to work around, not something that he will allow to limit him. There is no bravado in his attitude, no inflated sense of ego that makes him think he is indispensable. To the contrary, his words suggest that he knows he is rapidly dispensable and in a hurry to make a difference.

'What do your colleagues think?' I ask curiously, for this is not a situation one normally encounters.

His eyes grow serious. 'I think they are sad, but everyone tries to act normally when I am around. They have never made me feel uncomfortable although I am sure that takes work.'

'And how about the patients?' I am actually more fascinated to know the answer to this question. When patients are sick, they want their doctor to assume an even thicker cloak of invincibility. I know this from my own experience – lying in hospital, having lost the twins and feeling vulnerable, I wanted desperately to believe that my doctor knew all the answers; although when I was whole, I was under no illusion about this. There are lots of things that doctors do not know. There are lots of times when doctors do not feel well at work. How did Peter's patients react to the knowledge that their surgeon himself was damaged? In this small place, they had probably heard it on the grapevine that their surgeon was gravely ill. Did Peter tell the remaining patients? What happened if the chemotherapy-frayed nerves of Peter's fingers led him astray while performing crucial surgery? What words did Peter use to gain consent from patients to be operated on by him and did he hurt in the process?

'You know, patients are a gracious lot,' he says reflectively. 'And I feel great when I am operating, so that helps keep everyone's spirits up, mine included. The theatre is one place where I can leave my illness behind and concentrate on others. Of course, I wouldn't operate if I thought I was endangering lives, but I want to keep serving patients for as long as possible.' His eyes shine and light up his face as he talks about his patients.

I suddenly feel small. It is simply incredible that a sick man has the capacity, both physical and emotional, to stay engaged with his patients when he needs no excuse to bow out and concentrate on his own health. I am speechless at his courage, never really having met anyone like him. We talk for a little while longer and I am on the lookout to detect even a hint of self-pity or denial, finding neither. He simply acknowledges that like the thousands of patients he has treated, life has served him a severe blow. There is no arguing about its fairness or otherwise, he just wants to deal with what he has been given.

One of the nurses has taken my infant son for a walk while Peter and I talk. When she returns him to me, Peter exclaims in delight and asks to hold him. It is only when I reach out to hand him my son that we both remember that he is hooked to an IV pole. I hold my son on Peter's lap as he pulls a funny face. My toothless son giggles. Standing behind his chair, the nurse bites her lip and looks away. Suddenly conscious of tiring him out, I ask the nurse to take a few pictures of Peter and me. He poses gladly and smiles broadly in all of them. When it is time to leave, Peter reaches out to hug me.

'It was great to see you. Thank you for coming by.'

I hope my face does not reveal that this was an unplanned visit. Now, I deny even to myself that this is the last time I will see him. Numbed by sadness, I wish him luck. It does not escape me that he never once asks me a question or opinion related to his cancer. I am floored by his equanimity. I push my son's pram out before my tears start to run.

Back home, the pictures turn out well. I keep meaning to have extra copies printed to send to Peter, along with a note to say how much the meeting meant to me. But it seems too obvious and, I fear, somewhat priggish, so I hold back.

In the year that follows, I enquire about him from others at every opportunity. Each time the answer comes that things are slowly becoming worse. He continues to push himself at work but the days are getting harder as he grows unwell. There is unanimous agreement that he is a man who possesses uncommon willpower and unimaginable grace.

One day, I say aloud to a friend, 'You know, I have been meaning to write to Peter. Do you think he would even remember me?'

'Do it,' she urges. 'I think it would mean a lot to him.' I think that by expressing my intention aloud, I am committing myself to the deed. I even walk into the hospital card shop and cast around for an appropriate card, but leave empty-handed.

Then the inevitable occurs. While talking about another surgeon, a visiting friend mentions that Peter has died.

'Died?' I shriek, dismayed and dumbfounded. 'When? How?'

'You knew he had cancer, right?'

'Yes, yes, but no one told me he was dying!'

'He died two months ago.'

The news takes my breath away. Within minutes, I launch into a series of questions. Does she know how he died? Did he die at home with his devoted family at his side or did he spend his last days in a hospice? Was he still working? Could he speak and think towards the end? My friend does not have the answer to any of my questions and she does not note the urgency in my tone. She moves on to talk about other matters when all I want to do is find out more about how Peter died.

That evening, I call a second friend. 'I heard that Peter died.'

'Yes.'

'Do you know what happened?'

'Not a lot except he got very sick,' she answers. 'And it was a few months ago now, I can't really remember.'

But she leaves me with one tantalising detail. She tells me that Peter's funeral was packed and very moving and that the hospital had not felt the same for a long time afterwards. When I hang up, I never thought I could feel so sad or so left out of a life that I was only ever marginally involved in.

In the ensuing days, I roam the internet and old newspapers for details of Peter's life and death. I discover the charity he founded to support the poorest African communities, look at pictures of him operating by torchlight and sorting through donated medical aid. What is evident is his enthusiasm and empathy for people who he believed were worse off than him, not the cancer which he knows held him in its grip. I read that the cancer eventually travelled to his brain, curtailing his reserves but not his determination to make a difference. He kept up an active schedule, even leaving his hospital bed for engagements and travelling to Africa for a final involvement with the work his charity was performing. He spoke openly of his terminal illness and the desire to leave a meaningful legacy. I read personal memories and official obituaries – the plaudits seem to collect endlessly. They all celebrate his extraordinary life as a surgeon and mentor, but between the lines, the sadness of many who had lost more than a colleague is revealed. I can empathise, for despite my brief encounters with him, I feel as if I have lost a friend.

It seems strange and even intrusive to read so much about a man after his death that I could have discovered by talking to him during his life. It is as if I want to fill in the blanks without being found out. I wonder whether it was mere procrastination that prevented me from contacting Peter all those times I thought I should. Could I use my busy life – having had my second child by the time he died – as a legitimate excuse? For someone who is usually organised, neither explanation seems adequate. After all, I talk to cancer patients, some of whom are very sick, every day. I write condolence notes and make a host of phone calls, all without the slightest hesitation, considering it my obligation to do so.

I realise that what really prevented me from calling Peter is that his cancer felt too close to home. He was only in his mid-forties when first diagnosed, with a wife and young children. Being a doctor was not a mere job for him, but a calling, and when disease threatened to cut him off, he responded in the only way he knew, by continuing to give and serve. His profession anchored him – the students, doctors and patients he continued to engage with must have made him feel connected with the world, even as these connections grew tenuous. If I put myself in his place, my own instinct would be to do exactly as Peter did – fight a good and graceful fight, appreciating that many of my patients and their families face such tragedy, often with far fewer resources. I am just not sure whether I would be able to do it in his inimitable and admirable fashion.

Being the gifted doctor that he was, Peter could have recited verbatim the complications of his cancer. Did he lie awake at night worrying about which one would strike next? He would have known that patients often place the greatest faith in their doctor when there seems to be no other avenue of help. But he would appreciate equally that, in these instances, doctors can feel just as marooned as the patient. 'We will do everything we can' would have sounded so hollow to a doctor-turned-patient, well-versed in the limitations of medicine. Who did the reassurer turn to for reassurance?

Many months later, I hear from someone else that when conventional treatments failed him, he looked for experimental therapy. I wonder whether he approached these with trepidation and scepticism or his trademark fortitude and optimism. What happened when he became paralysed and wheelchair-bound, as someone had suggested? When his disease finally wrestled him away from his beloved profession, did he feel broken at last or lucky to have been given the grace of four years that many of his patients would not have had? I don't know. I will never know.

My silent relationship with Peter's illness continues. It is only now that I recognise that behind the silence lies a deep sadness that such an incomprehensible injustice could befall a good man. For all the inspiration he personified, his journey was terrifying and confronting. And sometimes, when faced with an overwhelming event, it seems safest just to watch from a distance. But the more I think about it, the more I acknowledge that my friend was right and that Peter, for all his strength, would have appreciated knowing how I felt about his plight. I know that had I just told him once, I would not live to regret all the occasions on which I came up short.

When I think of Peter, I think of writing to his family, but it seems far too late now. I console myself that of the hundreds of mourners gathered at his funeral and the thousands whose lives he touched, someone must have told him in person just how admired he was.

Dedicated to the memory of Peter Hewitt (1959–2008)

12

◇

It happens more than you think

She is halfway down my list of patients. The notes accompanying her name are short and look benign. 'Mrs Fernandez. Nice lady. Pain should be okay. Check infected needle site – better.' I allow myself to contemplate a good start to the weekend shift, which I am covering for a colleague on leave.

She is lying in her bed, a pink blanket laid neatly at her feet. She faces the busy, sunny road that lines the hospital; her body is half-turned, not sure about cooperating. A mop of shiny black hair adorns her petite head. She turns to look at me as I walk in. Her body is lithe and well-proportioned, well-tended despite her sixty years. She greets me warmly for a stranger and with an open attitude as she eases herself into a new position in bed. I notice the briefest wince before her smile wipes it away.

'I am the doctor looking after you this weekend.'

'Hello. I was expecting to see you,' she greets me back.

I am immediately enchanted by her dark brown, expressive eyes that set off her face like precious jewels. Her teeth are shiny, white, regular and intact. The nightgown, black and white, drapes grace-fully across her body, caressing its curves exactly as it is meant to.

Two broadsheet newspapers lie well-thumbed on the table. A pen rests beside a worn leather diary. Of the familiar signs of cancer – sympathy cards, flowers, photographs – there is none. I recheck my handover sheet to make sure she belongs in the oncology ward. 'Advanced disease, unknown primary tumour', the notes also say. She is looking up at me with anticipation. After the first ten patients, the checklist becomes automatic.

'How are you feeling this morning?'

'Not too bad.'

'Your pain?' She has bony metastases that are on the march.

'Okay.' She strokes her right cheek. 'The radiation will take a few days to work, I guess.'

'Are the painkillers causing side effects?'

'Less so now. I feel more awake on the reduced dose of morphine.'

'Anything I can do to help you today?'

I smile. She is the perfect patient. Well-controlled symptoms, understands her disease, on minimal medications, with a clear plan of action. She also recognises that I am filling in for her colleague and will defer questions for him. This is the moment of temptation every doctor feels to leave the room.

'No, I think I am just going to have a quiet day.'

I yield to the temptation but my conscience needles me as soon as my feet start back towards the door.

I haven't even sat down yet and she is finished. I look at my watch – it has taken two minutes so far. I can't leave like this. I try again.

'How are you doing emotionally?'

'How nice of you to ask! I think I am doing alright. I am quite okay.'

I should have guessed! This graceful, sensitive, 'with it' woman seems safely adjusted to her diagnosis. Her face is beguiling in its innocence, not a wrinkle on its landscape. She could probably teach the rest of us how to cope emotionally with what life deals us.

'Really?' I am running out of questions and starting to feel ridiculous. If I don't leave now, I suspect she will ask me if *I* am okay.

'Really.' I have heard this a hundred times before, with the response often hiding a private world of stoicism, resignation and built-up resistance to perceived gratuitousness. But I believe her. Her face is as peaceful as the statue of the Buddha that adorns a magazine cover on her bedside table. There is no doubting her answer.

A touch self-conscious but inwardly grateful, I prepare to move on to other patients. In leaving, I say, 'Well, I hope that you have a good weekend and get home soon.'

'Thank you, doctor.'

Her voice shimmers with amity and cooperation; it is mellifluous and puts one at ease. A patient like her every day or two would brighten the dreariest clinic. I like her, I think. I wonder what she is like and what she must have been like before her disease struck.

'Doctor, could you spare me an extra few minutes?'

I retrace my steps. Perhaps she has dropped her newspaper on the floor or wants me to chart some sleeping tablets or call her nurse. These are the usual things patients like her summon somebody back for.

'Are you from India?'

'Yes.'

'So am I! All these years and I still miss home.' Childlike eyes look up at me. But she couldn't have called me back simply to reminisce.

'I thought that since you asked how I was doing emotionally, I would tell you the truth. I want to talk to you about my condition.'

Her file states that she is a respected university professor who has worked at several places during her career. She is married with no children.

'I know that my cancer is bad and the fact that I have lived for two years is unexpected. After all, they gave me three months at diagnosis. It was very stable until recently but now it has started going to the bones.'

I read the results before coming in and agree with her that last week's bone scan lit up ominously. There were new metastases in her pelvis, sternum and vertebrae, but those exacting the greatest toll are the lesions in the base of her skull, ambushing nerves at their exit and causing pain hard to describe and harder to treat. Morphine makes her somnolent and she complains of feeling drugged. She has recently received radiation therapy for severe pain in her jaw, but now she has developed facial nerve involvement. This is a crucial nerve that commands movement of the face as well as the faculty of taste. She describes the sensation of the malfunctioning nerve eloquently, as that of a feather tickling her throat as she eats spoilt food.

She squares herself in her bed, looks me in the eye and says, 'I don't want to die with one nerve going after the other. I know that many important nerves travel through the skull.'

Her fear tallies with my own so I reassure us both. 'The radiotherapy will do a good job of controlling your pain and prevent further complications.'

'But you can't cure the cancer.'

I prick my ears to gauge whether this is a statement or a question, but it's too late. Far too many patients report that they have never been told that their cancer is incurable. But they say this to people other than their oncologist: some patients are reluctant to ask, others are afraid to know while yet others assume that their oncologist will somehow find a way to convey the unwelcome message. The oncologist who does not explicitly tell does so to avoid sowing further seeds of sorrow, but silently hopes that there is enough in the nuance of his words and actions that makes clear his fears for the patient. Thus patient and doctor exist in a fog, each feeling uncomfortable with what the other does not know.

Cautiously, I enquire, 'What does your oncologist say?'

'He says there is nothing else he can do. But he is very nice,' she then hastens to add.

'I am afraid more chemotherapy would not be useful but there is room for painkillers and radiation.' I am relieved that all I have to do is agree with her oncologist.

'Can I talk to you unofficially?' she suddenly asks, looking even more alert.

It is an odd request but she looks expectant.

'I am your doctor today and you can certainly talk to me,' I offer, my curiosity getting the better of me.

'When you asked me how I am doing emotionally, I said okay. And I am for now. But the more I think about it, the more afraid I am of the indignity of this slow death. I am always in pain. First one bone, then the next; first one nerve, then another. Unable to open my mouth properly, unable to taste, then to swallow, speak, have a conversation with my family. I am not complaining about life's unfairness but I just don't want to live like this when things get worse. And we both know they will.'

Her words compel me to smell her fear, a rational one. In my mind's eye, I see her cancer cells on a determined march through her body.

'Maybe the radiation will stabilise things for quite some time.'

She detects my noncommittal tone and responds earnestly. 'But think about it. The nasty thing is spreading. It will spring up elsewhere, perhaps next inside my brain. I don't want to live like this.'

It is indeed remarkable that she has come so far but the trajectory of her illness is now obvious. She has failed various lines of conventional as well as complementary therapy and in the last few weeks has become increasingly troubled by her symptoms.

'I am not saying that I would, but how can I end it if it is no longer a life I want to lead?' She fixes me with an unflinching stare.

The sharp drawing in of my breath echoes through the spacious room. My heart pounds. In a flash, I am distressed, concerned, confused and flustered.

'I am not *that* kind of a doctor!' I want to counter indignantly, ending the conversation there and then. Her eyes, steeled with courage, have lost none of their charm. Her expression too is disarmingly soft. I can hear every part of her thinking, anticipating, preparing for my next words. She gently taps the luminous silver dial of her watch in a practised motion she must have performed before her students hundreds of times.

'My entire family has placed its life on hold, and now we are all waiting for the clock to strike twelve. Eventually, there isn't going to be any quality left in this waiting. Is it so wrong to want to go before then?'

I am stunned by her cold logic yet captivated by its lucidity. She is thinking aloud what has crossed the minds of anyone, doctor or patient, who has witnessed the trail of emotional and physical destruction that a terminal illness often lays down. I immediately think about all the times that I, along with my colleagues, have expressed our thoughts with statements like, 'I don't blame her for wanting to die', or 'I am glad he is finally gone', our words belying our frustrated acknowledgement that sometimes the best symptom relief we offer is still not good enough for the patient who mourns the loss of quality of life. But the comments are strictly private, spoken in careful asides, well-shielded from our public personas, which are charged with maintaining hope, counselling courage.

I respond firmly. 'Physician-assisted suicide is illegal. I am afraid I can't help you.'

She sighs. 'I know and I understand. I just hate losing control over this final aspect of my life that affects all those around me.'

'Does your husband know your wishes?'

A knock on the door makes me jump. I assume that someone has been listening and my entire mien assumes a guilty appearance although I have done nothing wrong. Her husband walks in and strokes her hair before shaking my hand. I feel distinctly awkward that I have been talking about his wife's death behind his back.

'Have a seat,' she tells him. 'We have just been discussing that same thing.'

'Oh yes,' he says briskly and warmly. 'And does the doctor have any ideas?'

'What sort of people are they?' my mind screams. They refer to death as if it were a mere blood count or another prescription for antibiotics.

'Physician-assisted suicide is illegal,' I restate more loudly than necessary. I need to hear myself say it because I also need to say what comes next: 'I can see that you are fearful about your future.' In fact, in her fear, I sense a vestige of the same existential question that gnaws at many of us, ill and well. What would we want if we were destined to die a slow and painful death? Would we favour survival over quality and what would tilt us in which direction? Who could we entrust with respecting our final wish if it were the most important we had ever desired?

She seizes my statement of sympathy as a breathless man clutches at oxygen. 'You understand my fear because you have seen lives become untenable. You *know* I am right.' Subtle accusation and stern conviction are finely mixed in the statement, so gently delivered yet hitting hard. I have often felt uncomfortable but never so insecure in the presence of a patient. I feel powerless, swimming hard against a mighty current but partially tempted to just succumb to it. I recoil at the horror of even contemplating euthanasia because it goes against the grain of everything I was taught as a doctor – to heal, to care, to ease suffering. To hasten death? All I ever learnt while training was that it was decried by the jury of one's peers and punishable by law. But then, why can I not dismiss outright her request as absurd? Why do I find her argument compelling? Because in her reasoning, I see shades of my own. There is a power differential between us today but it is easy to imagine myself in her shoes, begging for what she wants.

'Tell me, doctor, have you met many patients with incurable cancer?'

'Yes.' It is the easiest of today's questions.

'And how many have asked you to help them die?'

'None,' I respond, knowing that this is not technically correct as some patients have, but never as deliberately as her, thus allowing me to explore other factors in their request such as untreated pain, depression, guilt and anger.

'Are you depressed?' I enquire of her gently. 'I know you have had a rough time recently. I could find you someone to talk to. In fact, we have an excellent psychiatrist.'

'I am not depressed,' she says, without taking umbrage. 'Like many rational people, I want to plan ahead. You just have to believe me.'

I believe her entirely.

Her husband has been watching the street bustling with traffic and people. He picks up the newspaper and, pretending to scan it, muses, 'You know, it happens more commonly out there than you think.'

His statement sears me. How far advanced are their plans and what is my obligation to her and to my profession?

'How are you going to achieve what you want?' I am not sure what I will do with the knowledge and I secretly hope that she does not divulge any more. But I have asked the question and they seem unafraid to answer it.

'I think I will fly to a country where it is easier. Luckily, we know doctors around the world. We both agree we don't want to cause trouble.' She says this with utter frankness, as if negotiating a minor traffic impediment. Then she looks into the street before sighing. 'But what a shame I can't die in the comfort of my own house where I have lived the best part of my life. Every room soothes me and simply being home feels like good medicine. You might laugh, but sometimes I forget my pain just by sitting in the garden that I have tended over thirty years.' It is this devastating normalisation that makes her sound like any one of us.

The conversation comes to a natural halt. I don't know what else to say and they don't feel the need to continue. The more peaceful their demeanour, the more churned up I feel. It is as if I have done wrong by simply sanctioning this conversation yet I know that her mind was made up well before she met me and that I was nothing more than a sounding board. I even feel irked at the thought that I have been a mere pawn in their well-hatched plan to end her life on her terms. The modern doctor is meant to walk step in step with the patient, part guardian of health, but increasingly a service provider. Guidelines abound to help us become sound practitioners but what are the rules when the practice is death? Is assisted death always unconscionable for being a dereliction of our duty to first do no harm? Or is it, like virtually all other procedures and practices, one that is nuanced? And if so, can I trust myself to weigh the nuances with the sagacity and deliberation that this irrevocable act demands?

In the doctor's entry for the day, I write benignly, 'Overall not too bad. Keen to get home. Pain management still needs fine-tuning.' I am struck by how easy it is to subvert the truth. Although I try to convince myself that I am writing only this brief note to protect her privacy, I know that it also reflects my sense of impotence.

What do I do for patients like her? I wonder. Do I dismiss out of hand their call for assistance beyond that which I am capable of or willing to provide? Or do I subject myself to deep soul-searching at the cost of creating chaos within myself? If the conscience is torn between professional obligation and personal conviction, will the profession find it in its heart to counsel and comfort or will it disown those who venture into the unknown?

I wonder about her from time to time but intentionally avoid calling her oncologist to follow up on her progress, fearing that the news can only be bad. I am also conscious that I may be the only person she has divulged her secret to and don't want to place her in an awkward situation.

One day, about six weeks later, her husband suddenly calls.

'I hope you don't mind me calling you.'

'No, no, I don't.' What could he possibly want from me?

'My wife is still alive but in a lot more pain. I don't know who to ask without arousing suspicion, but will the airlines let her fly?'

Fear strikes my heart.

'Where do you want to take her?'

'Out of here.'

I take his not so subtle hint.

'I am sorry, but how can I say? I only met your wife once and that was weeks ago. Have you spoken to her oncologist about this?'

'No. I don't know that he would be impressed. He has really tried hard with her.'

'Depending on how sick your wife is, the airline may need a doctor's letter and it would have to be from someone who is treating her.'

'Oh, really?'

'Has she made up her mind to go?'

'You know, her greatest desire is to die at home. But how can I say it – death just will not come.' His voice contains equal measures of grief and exasperation. 'What does it take for someone to die? What is so meaningful or memorable about her suffering? It is so unfair.'

'Try talking to your oncologist,' I urge. 'You may be surprised at what he can do to help.'

'I don't see that happening.'

'I am sorry. I wish there was something I could do to help you both.'

'Thank you for your time, doctor. It's okay.'

What did he *really* call me for, I ask myself. Surely, they are both intelligent enough to recognise that I am not in a position to clear her to fly. Did they think I had an alternative solution? Did they suspect that her predicament had bothered me enough to rethink my position? I don't know whether to feel complimented or rattled by their implied trust in me.

But when I contemplate her sobering future, my self-indulgence melts and I see that why I am so bothered by the entire conversation is because my negative response to her initial request was visceral in its intensity. No, I had stated firmly, I could not help her die. Perhaps I would be concerned if the response were anything but; however, what troubles me is that I did not find her argument unreasonable or worthy of dissuasion. I was only grateful that I could obscure my haplessness by quoting the law. But how much longer will my respite last? As medicine continues its impressive onslaught on diseases and the population hobbles towards an older age, we are destined to find ourselves delivering quantity but not always quality of life. When the sheer burden of such a life wearies our patients and some seek to end it, their doctors will face the question more often than they might like to think. At issue of course is not only what is medically appropriate but the interplay with law, politics and religion. I am not sure that we will agree in our own lifetime but what matters most is not to turn away from the problem and continue to address it with the sensitivity and honesty our patients deserve.

From time to time I wonder if this was my final conversation with her husband. I am astonished when he phones me again many weeks later, just as I thought I would never hear from him again.

'I thought it was only fair to fill you in.'

I feel like a child being offered a dangerous temptation. I suspect that it may not be good for me but just then, I desperately want it, without paying heed to its ramifications.

'How is she?' I ask.

'She finally died last week.'

I quickly calculate that it took her nearly three months to die after our first meeting and feel sorry for her suffering. There was nothing wrong with her wishing to do away with the savage pain at the end of her life.

'I am sorry for your loss.'

'This is not meant to sound cruel but her death could not have come soon enough.'

I gather from his statement that their plans for euthanasia did not materialise.

He fills me in: 'She wanted to fly out but felt too deeply attached to our house to leave. This is a house that has been in her family since she was a child. She was religious and believed that her soul would go in peace if she died there.'

'Was she comfortable?'

'No. No matter what we tried, she just never got comfortable.'

'The drugs didn't help?'

'They helped a little but she said that her real pain was the pain of her helplessness,' he replies.

Her description hit the nail on the head again. Like her husband, my predominant feeling at her passing is one of relief.

'I am very sorry. I only met her once but she sounded like good company.'

'The real reason I am calling is because she told me to. She thought that you gave her the chance to think aloud and she always wondered whether she had taken undue liberty of your willingness to listen. She told me she felt bad for putting you on the spot but you gave her your ear, which was more than she expected.'

'I didn't mind at all,' I lie.

'Thank you. She would have been relieved to hear that.'

I sigh inwardly. Not everyone has the capacity to be so gracious and thoughtful while dealing with their own death. Without even knowing her, I mourn her loss to the human fraternity.

Our conversation ends like countless others.

'If you ever want to talk about this some more, you know how to reach me. Please don't hesitate to call.'

'Yes, doctor, I know. Thank you.'

'Goodbye.'

That was two years ago.

13

◇

You have to help me

'You have to help me,' she urges. Her warmth penetrates the sterility of my windowless office. She is simply beautiful. Despite the cancer that is said to be consuming her from the inside.

Those fluid brown eyes, with long black lashes for a guard, speak a language of their own. Her complexion is impeccable, as if molten honey was smoothed over her skin at birth in a single master stroke. Her eyebrows, shaped in a perfect arch, travel up ever so slightly as she opens her mouth to speak, revealing sparkling, white teeth framed by full lips with barely a hint of gloss. Were she to smile, it would captivate a room many times as large as mine. She is far too beautiful to have cancer, I decide.

'You have to help me,' she repeats, waking me from my reverie.

I look down at her file, which I have just picked up for the first time. She is a new patient to the hospital clinic, having transferred her care to us after being given bad news elsewhere. A summary from her previous oncologist outlines her diagnosis at the age of thirty. She had presented with a persistent cough at a time when her entire family had developed a cold. Her family doctor reassured her it was a viral infection, the after effects of which could take several weeks to settle. Weeks later, when her family was well and she felt worse, she took herself back to the doctor and got a chest X-ray. The X-ray revealed lung cancer.

She began treatment with chemotherapy within a week of the diagnosis, and within three months many of the spots had disappeared and the remaining ones had shrunk. The oncologist called this one of the most gratifying responses he had ever witnessed. In remission, she enjoyed a good quality of life. However, the letter went on to say, nine months later, a routine scan showed tumour progression. She began treatment and again responded well, although somewhat less completely. The second remission was also not as long. Within two months, she was feeling worse and the scans reflected this. The cancer had spread beyond the lungs and the oncologist advised her that she stood to benefit little from further treatment. She did not return to him.

Despite the failure of multiple treatments, I am surprised at how well she presents today. If she feels as well as she looks, I can understand why she would not wish to entertain the thought of there being no further treatment for her cancer.

'Isn't there anything?' Her husband's face is contorted in a plea.

An open wallet peeking from her bag reveals a family picture, a relic of happier times. I avert my eyes.

'Tell me a little about yourself,' I say.

He holds her hand and she repeats the story. But she adds that she is the mother of three young children, between seven and four years of age. She tells me that they fled war-torn Sri Lanka to forge a new life for the family. Like many young couples, they led a parsimonious existence in the beginning. He had been an engineer back home but attended night school to gain new qualifications.

With her professional skills and pleasant manner, she was offered a job as a secretary but went on to become the personal assistant to a prominent barrister.

'Our life was finally on track when this happened,' he grimaces.

Lives interrupted in their element – this is the way it frequently seems to be.

We look through her most recent scans together and I point out the major abnormalities. I am silently shocked by the extent of her cancer, recognising that her apparent well-being is temporary. I tell her that my reading of her situation is as pessimistic as my colleague's but I would be happy to see her.

'I want to have more treatment,' she says. 'I want to do everything I can.'

Her single-minded approach to treatment is understandable. That cancer is an inconvenience to be rooted out of a busy life at any cost is a trait I most commonly observe in young parents struck unexpectedly by the disease. They convey the attitude that their hours are so filled with packing lunch boxes and ferrying the children that they don't even have time to contemplate being jolted out of their hectic if predictable life. I would counsel many patients to forego such treatment for the sake of quality of life but she has already indicated that for her, quality equates to extent of life.

'Every day I can open my eyes is another day I can see my children.'

He looks on silently.

The chemotherapy is associated with many hiccups. In the intervals when she should be home recovering, she is often in hospital, receiving a blood transfusion, being examined for a fever, having more scans. She begins to lose weight and the glow on her face when I first saw her seems dulled, but she keeps coming back for more.

'Are you sure you want to keep going?'

'Yes. I don't have a choice.'

You *do* have a choice, I would insert at some point, to someone else, but when I go to say these words to her, I am reminded of my own son. I know what she means.

She never formally stops chemotherapy but the development of a pleural effusion – fluid trapped between the lining of the lung – leads to a series of deferments. One day in clinic she arrives unable to breathe. I admit her to the ward where two litres of fluid are drained from her left lung, causing instant relief. 'I didn't know the lung could hold so much fluid,' she remarks, able to take her first deep breaths. Unfortunately, as she will discover, it can hold multiples of this amount. After three drainage procedures in quick succession, she submits to surgery to stick the lining together to prevent accumulation of fluid. Her breathing improves but the disruption of nerves in the region leads to significant pain. Out of hospital on her own insistence because she wants to be with her children, she lets me chase her pain. The attempt is dashed from the start. Morphine makes her drowsy and unable to drive the children or even be attentive to their conversation at home. Steroids cause her dormant reflux symptoms to reappear. Other drugs just don't work. She is miserable with pain.

'Can I admit you to hospital and ask our pain team to help?' I ask woefully.

'No, I am spending too much time in hospital as it is, doctor. Can't *you* do something more?'

I spend hours discussing her case with anaesthetists all over town. They quiz me about her cancer and her prognosis. They read the reports and shake their head. 'You have to meet her before you decide,' I appeal to the most experienced one. I am sure that her personal reasons are more compelling than the dismal course of her cancer. To my surprise he agrees, and to my relief, he decides to offer her a complicated treatment.

'I have told her that the main risks of a nerve block in this area are that one, it may not work and two, it could lead to her permanent paralysis.'

She returns wondering which unenviable choice to make. We spend another few weeks adjusting her pain relief although it feels to me as if we are simply shuffling cards. She eventually concludes that anything would be better than tolerating the continuous and excruciating pain in her chest. Terrified about the prospect of being admitted to yet another hospital with its bevy of strangers, she keeps her calm by concentrating on the procedure and the kindly anaesthetist who is performing it. Afterwards, she feels distinctly better, though not pain-free, and asks to be discharged home within twenty-four hours. Her husband calls me to report that she has not felt like this in months. I pray that the situation lasts forever.

She returns to have more chemotherapy. I observe that she never expresses an exaggerated claim of what she hopes this will achieve; for her, the mere fact of dragging herself to another day in the chemotherapy chair is testament to her determination to fight. I feel more despondent than ever at the prospect of more chemotherapy, fearful that it will lead to a fatal complication. I hint at this.

'I can't die. My children need me,' she says, ending the conversation.

Tragically, I am saved from filling out her chemotherapy prescription by a diagnosis that same evening of a tumour in her brain. After neurosurgery, she is fast asleep and does not notice me standing at her bedside. Her wrapped head makes her look ill and vulnerable. The notes say that the surgery went well. Since the operation, she has spoken fluently and moved all her limbs. So well, in fact, that the next time I call in, she is gone. Her doctor exclaims that this was one of the speediest recoveries he has seen in a cancer patient. 'She must have an amazing constitution,' he enthuses. Or very young children who rely on her.

When she returns to see me, the most noticeable change in her is that she is wearing her hair in a short crop. 'They took part of it away at surgery so I decided to cut it,' she said.

Many women have said that they find losing their hair the most distressing and confronting aspect of their entire treatment, for once their hair goes, they are announcing their disease to the world, inviting along with it many sidelong glances and sympathetic utterances. Suddenly cancer invades their bus journey to work, the children's pick-up from school and the supermarket checkout that had always been routine.

'Can I have more treatment?'

'I am running out of ideas.'

'You have to help me! There is nobody else.'

She is thirty-two, dying. I am thirty-two, charged with saving her. The more desperate she becomes, the less I deliver. She sits awkwardly in the cramped waiting room, holding up a tired body and a worn spirit. She must have memorised every gossip magazine in the room and read every sign a hundred times, so she just stares at her hands now, looking up only when I say her name. She must think she is just another person down the list, though her young age and vulnerable situation make her anything but. In truth, I sometimes wish I had the luxury of spending the entire morning sifting through her issues, which are multiplying with time. But part of the art of medicine lies in exercising good judgement *with* compassion in *finite* time. I find that I have to remind myself that each patient who is waiting outside has his own personal tragedy unfolding – I just happen to know more about hers. I find the reminder distasteful but necessary to maintain objectivity.

Over the months, I have grown to admire her resilience. Most days I struggle to hide my dismay at her worsening state and if I am sometimes a little forceful in my assertion that we have exhausted our options, it is because I want to avoid injecting false hope. She regards me as her saviour but when the door closes behind her, I question the existence of a god more crudely and intensely than she. I run into a chaplain whom I have known since my days as a student and I tell him this. The chaplain says it is important to have faith but his words sound hollow. Week after week, her prayers and mine go unanswered. She weeps. I feel terrified.

On a subsequent appointment her five-year-old daughter holds her hand as she heaves into a bowl. Can she sense my scant reassurance? My heart aches as I instinctively think of my own son, confident that I will return home to him.

Different doctors dislike different aspects of their job. My greatest dislike is watching patients vomit. There is something about the very defencelessness of already beaten bodies that I find deeply upsetting. My mother recollects that when I misbehaved as a child, she only had to tell me she felt sick and I would be subdued. This trait, professionally not the most helpful, has only become more ingrained with time.

'You have to let me admit you!' I shout over the sound of her vomiting. 'You can't possibly go home like this!' I look away. Too sick to argue, she simply nods, tears streaming down her face, oblivious to my company.

I watch helplessly as she is wheeled away, crying in agony, a wounded animal. 'We will make her better,' I whisper to her daughter. Mutual desolation fills the air.

'Last night, we waited so long in emergency,' her husband says, accusation and grief merging into one. What I wouldn't do to return to her those needlessly spent eight hours, revisiting the painful details of her sentence. I hand him my mobile phone number. It is my way of saying I will do anything to make her numbered days more bearable.

'I will try any drug, however toxic,' she beseeches on the ward.

In her absence, I scour the literature, ask the experts. There is nothing. Surrounded by advice, I feel lost in the wilderness of an incurable disease.

Why did I become a doctor? To heal the suffering of others, not to observe from the sidelines a young life brazenly plundered. What is the point of witnessing the agony of patients? Guilt and venom wash over me, and then unrelenting sorrow at the sheer futility of my position as I preside over her untimely death. How will I move on? Is it even conceivable to reconcile with this injustice?

Soon she is in hospice. I visit her every day. The palliative care doctors and nurses are kind and attentive, but I can't shirk my moral obligation. Sometimes, finding her asleep, I steal away unnoticed, guilty but grateful for the respite from confronting both her death and my impotence. Then, the drawings of her children arrest me, brightness forced on a bleak landscape. One day, as the weather grows warmer, I park my car on the street and walk briskly to the hospice. By the time I enter her room, I have broken into a fine sweat. I eagerly throw off my trench coat, revealing the full bloom of a pregnancy that I have managed to conceal from her so far.

'Oh! I didn't know you were having a baby!'

I am mortified at the thoughtless juxtaposition of life and death in the making. But with clouded eyes and a shaking voice, she congratulates me warmly, saying that she knows I will make a good mother.

'*You* are a good mother,' I tell her honestly. It is too difficult to think through the nuances of telling the truth. Outside, I weep, wondering how any world design could include wrenching mother from child.

She fades away, her pleas drying on parched lips. One day, she whispers, 'Help me die so I don't have to think about losing the children anymore.' Her words fall like blows. Far from distancing myself from her plight, I feel broken imagining it. I hold her hand in silence, quivering at the horror of her circumstances, but am stunned when I too find myself hoping she dies soon. I want to slip away into an abyss of darkness where I can violently shake off her very memory. Conflict fills my head. I hate the idea of being her doctor, no longer sure whether I am helping or hurting. What is essential about this experience for either of us?

'I can't hasten your death,' I say, 'but I won't abandon you.' I am ashamed at the courage I must summon to say this.

A few days later, I have to leave for a conference. I had expected her to die before my departure but she hangs on. I tell her I will be away for a few days.

'Maybe you will come back with a new idea,' she says.

New ideas take decades to translate into drugs. She doesn't need to know that.

She is on my mind for the duration of the conference, but when I return, the pending work doesn't permit me to see her for the first few days. When I finally get to the hospice, the intern says, 'She has been asking for you every day but we told her that you were uncontactable.'

I stare at her in disbelief. 'Why would you do that? You knew I was back.'

'She just doesn't want to believe that there is no other treatment. I figured you would be sick of telling her the same thing.'

I bite my tongue, forcing myself to think that the intern doesn't know any better, that in keeping with her training to become self-sufficient, she was only trying to protect me, the person who doesn't need protecting.

'Next time, let me make that decision.'

Inside, the patient's eyes light up for a moment when I enter.

'I knew you would come back!'

When I find my voice, I turn to her husband to apologise. She returns to a sedated sleep.

'Oh, don't worry,' he says. 'I just told her that each time you came by, she was sleeping. It was less distressing.' His eyes are red from lack of rest and constant worry.

She dies after clinging to life by a seemingly endless thread. She denies pain to avoid more sedation. She feigns strength to smile at her children. She still asks about experimental treatments. Then she sinks back, defeated. Silently I curse her fate, struggling alongside her in her tortured journey. My faith in medicine melts before this testing spectacle.

He calls me after her funeral. One of the desk clerks took the time to go and she has filled me in on the details. The people at the service spilled over from the church onto the streets. The eulogies spoke of the difference she had made in the lives of others, especially new migrants. Her children sat quietly, not quite sure what to make of the crowd. Her husband stayed close to them, busily moving his eyes from one to the next. Everywhere, there was a thick cover of disbelief. I am infinitely relieved to have missed the funeral.

My colleagues console me, saying the therapies failed her and her body betrayed her. But somewhere in our journey, her fears, hopes and desires merged with mine and I feel an abject failure. When my daughter is born and my birthday arrives, I suffer a form of survival guilt. Her death is the closest I have ever come to reconsidering my career as an oncologist. In the silence of my morning walks, I reflect on a change in career, tempted by the notion of witnessing a little less sadness and failure while still performing the task of a doctor. There is no shame in protecting myself and my family from the cloud of intense emotion that I unwittingly cast over us all from time to time. But somehow, I keep returning to the thought that to leave oncology would be giving up. Giving up on the teachers who took such pains to teach me, on the patients who need me, but most of all, giving up on myself, unable to translate a profoundly distressing experience into anything more than a fear of having to repeat it. By leaving, I could relinquish the right to observe as keenly that as the science of medicine advances, its art must not be abandoned. For nowhere is the art of medicine more wanted than in the cancer clinic. Patients do not have a choice in the matter of their disease. Having chosen to accompany them, it seems unfair to opt out because the journey is more arduous than I thought.

She leaves me a note. It takes me a long time to open it. I hesitate mainly because I am not yet ready to face her recriminations from the grave. I don't need to read about it to know that I let her down. Instead, it is almost as if she comes alive saying the words: 'Thank you for listening.'

I am amazed, humbled beyond words. I tell myself that if her memory helps me realise what is really important about being a doctor – honesty, partnership and compassion – for the rest of my career, her death may yet yield some meaning.

14

◇

I'm doing what's right for me

'I will think about it,' he says, shaking his head.

I turn my head curiously. 'I am sorry?'

'I said I will think about it.'

'So you are still not sure?'

'No.'

'You know, I hate to labour the point . . .'

'Then don't.'

'Okay, I hear you, Mr Ambrose.'

'Good. So will you still see me?'

'If you want me to.'

'I might have to think about that too, but for now I will make an appointment.'

He rises from his chair and walks across the length of the room, clutching his side. Her eyes uncertainly follow him, then me. When he is close, she tugs at a corner of his jacket and makes a questioning gesture with her hand. He barks at her in a foreign language. She shrinks back into her chair and I can feel my hackles rise. He gathers his belongings, takes the appointment slip and opens the door. She follows meekly.

He is seventy-eight years old. She must be no more than thirty. 'Your typical mail-order bride,' someone sniggered earlier. I look at her diminutive figure and shrug. It is none of our business.

He was getting the groceries when he collapsed in the aisle with pain. He had always been well and played golf until three years ago when his failing vision forced him off the course. He told the paramedics that it was probably a stomach spasm and he would be fine, but they took him to hospital. The doctors found blood in his urine and a large cancerous tumour in his kidney. Judging by its size, it was remarkable that it had not caused any symptoms before.

I was called to see him on the ward. He was receiving a blood transfusion when I knocked on his door. He looked wan and uncomfortable so we did not talk long. I introduced myself, checked that he was aware of the diagnosis, and offered to tell him more. But he demurred, just wanting to get out of hospital. Most patients can recall little of what they are told in hospital so I acquiesced to seeing him in clinic.

'Do you have any family to bring with you?'

'Yes, my wife.'

'Good. Two pairs of ears are better than one.'

Today, I cannot help but notice what a difference normal clothes make to the appearance of even the most rundown patient. Contrary to the earlier impression I had of him, he looks surprisingly robust for his age, a legacy of a healthy and active life. He had been a promising athlete in school and ran his last marathon at the age of sixty-five.

'I had to get a doctor's certificate before they would let me run!' he recalls proudly.

We talk about his diagnosis and he asks a number of questions. I explain that his biopsy confirms the diagnosis of cancer. 'However, the good news is that your scans show that it is contained. The surgeons can take it out by removing the kidney.'

I pause for the usual patient response to this kind of news – exclamations of surprise followed by relief. Instead, he says, 'We'll see about that.'

Just to be sure, I repeat myself. 'I think your cancer is curable with surgery.'

'We'll see.' His expression is deadpan.

I am puzzled by his attitude. Does he not understand or has he not heard me? For a man who has just provided an expansive account of his life, this sudden veneer of inscrutability leaves me confounded. I look at his wife, who has not moved since she sat down. She regards him deferentially but I am not sure how much of the conversation she has understood. His attitude makes it clear that she is not his equal in this dialogue so I desist from addressing her directly.

'I will just write some notes as you have a think about things.' I know that this interval of seconds is woefully small but, frankly, I didn't think he would need even this. After all, what does one have to weigh when faced with the commutation of a death sentence?

When I look up, his face is still wooden, his thoughts paused. I feel a faint stir of impatience.

'So what would you like to do?'

'Give me another appointment.'

'Okay. I will see you next week.' Some patients need longer than others to come to terms with their circumstances. Perhaps his unexpected reprieve has shocked him to such an extent that he doesn't know how to respond. Maybe he is not as stoic as he thought. I give him an appointment slip. She looks at him quizzically but does not say anything. He ushers her out with a hand on the small of her back.

When he returns, he brings a surprise with him. It is his son, about five years old, a blend of his father's complexion and his mother's peaceable expression.

He looks around inquisitively, intrigued by the pink handwash on the sink.

'What's your name, young man?' I smile as I offer him a squirt of the handwash.

His head peeps shyly from behind his mother.

'It's Thomas,' his father offers.

'He is beautiful,' I say instinctively. She is clearly delighted with the appraisal.

Thomas behaves impeccably throughout the consultation while his father asks me questions that are very similar to last week's. We cover the same basic ground again. I touch on the complications of an anaesthetic and the potential implications of losing one kidney, although I expect him to manage well on the remaining one. I explain that the surgeon will detail the operation when he sees him.

'When I finish, I will call the surgeon. He's nice, you will like him,' I say encouragingly.

'Excuse me, doctor,' he says before turning to his wife. She immediately collects Thomas and goes outside.

'I don't want to have any treatment.'

'What?'

'I don't want to have an operation.'

'Why is that?'

'Because I don't want to.' He shrugs and looks straight ahead at the wall.

I take a deep breath. 'This is an aggressive cancer. It will take your life.'

'I guess we all have to die of something.'

Spare me the cliché, I silently groan.

'Having a kidney taken out is not the most major of operations. We could talk to your surgeon about the ways in which this could be done, so you get home quickly.' I feel uncomfortable, as if I am lying under oath. I ought to know that for the person destined to go under the knife, there is no such clear distinction between operations. Doctors, not patients, use the term 'minor surgery'. I remember the fury I felt when I was taken to theatre for a procedure following the loss of my twins. Although it fulfilled its medical description of being necessary, painless and quick, I found the entire episode simply terrifying and the memory of my loss of control still freezes me.

'I don't want to have it.' His voice is calm, without a hint of challenge.

'But why not?' I sound like a petulant teenager asking for permission to go out at night.

'I don't want to.' He is the equally unrelenting parent, not interested in explaining his reasons.

I stop to try a different, less confrontational tactic.

'It is common and natural to be scared of surgery. Do you think you feel this way?'

'No, I have broken a leg before on the ski slopes and had to be rushed to emergency theatre to have six hours of surgery.' Thus he extinguishes my line of reasoning.

'Perhaps I have made the operation sound more complicated than it is. I am sure you will find the surgeon easier to follow – he does this regularly.'

'I think you explained it pretty clearly, actually.'

'Then is there something else I have missed?'

'No.'

I am about to resume the entire line of questioning when I suddenly stop in my tracks. I am trying to convince a man to accept treatment for cancer! In the microcosm of diseases which I preside over, the clashes, controversies and bargaining take place over having more treatment and extending life, not refusing a cure! On occasion people have declined treatment and I have assented, for we both know that they have been rendered so sick and disabled by their disease that chemotherapy would only add to their battle. I can't think of anybody who has refused potentially curative surgery. On the contrary, the mere mention of cancer unleashes a desperate drive in most individuals to be rid of it, even if the chances of success do not seem great. Patients still place tremendous faith in the ability of the knife to cure, and a substantial portion of my time is spent gently undoing the fixed determination of patients with advanced cancer that their cure lies in the fingers of an expert surgeon.

'Are you sure they can't just take it out?' is one of the most frequent questions I am asked. Patients are awestruck by surgeons. But here, finally, is a man who simply refuses to believe the true claim that a surgeon can cure him. I am fascinated.

The temporary silence that has fallen between us is interrupted by an insistent knock.

'You can come in,' he permits, allowing himself a brief smile.

His wife and son sit down quietly.

'So then, doctor, we are finished, right?'

I am nonplussed by the superficial exchange. But I push my chair back from the desk, holding my hands up, mildly annoyed at myself for trying so hard.

'Yes, we are.'

In spite of my secret wish that he not return and instead be consigned to that group of patients who we simply lose track of but wonder what happened to, he adheres to all his appointments. He comes alone, armed with a coffee in one hand and a newspaper in the other, prepared to wait. A man who clearly cares about his appearance, he always wears clean, pressed clothes and is freshly shaved. Looking at him in the waiting room, one would never guess that he is anything other than the conventional patient.

Our conversations always start off the same way. He tells me about the morning's terrible traffic run followed by a discourse on a different country's public transport system each time until I feel rather like an armchair expert on buses and trains. Then I enquire about his symptoms. The pain in his abdomen has never really gone away completely. At first, he avoided accepting any painkillers but recently he has quickly gone up the ladder of drugs to morphine. However, he resists changing doses frequently and flatly refuses to come into hospital for pain management.

'It is quite unsatisfactory treating your pain like this because I don't see you often enough. I am sure I could do a better job if you were an inpatient.'

'No thanks. I would rather spend time with my son.'

This mention of his son needles me.

'Can I get the palliative care nurses to see you at home?'

'No. My wife attends to my every need. I don't know what I would do without her.'

Does he ever ponder the reverse, I can't help wondering. What will his timid, non-English speaking wife do when he is no more? Will his death extinguish her dream of a better life for herself and their son?

Since the time he made his intentions clear, I have not raised the question of surgery again but I keep my ears pricked for even the slightest suggestion on his part that he is reconsidering. He seems a proud man and I stand ready to ease the process should he just say the word. But not only is he a proud man, he is also a steadfast one.

One day, fresh from speaking to a psychiatrist colleague, I say, 'You know, sometimes we find that unrecognised depression can lead people to hesitate in making decisions about cancer treatment. I am not claiming that you are depressed but would you like to speak a psychiatrist to explore this?'

It is his turn to study me.

'Do you think I am depressed?'

'You don't appear to be,' I admit. 'But depression may not be obvious.'

'Do you have concerns about my decision-making capacity?'

I am surprised by his turn of phrase but realise that he has probably looked into the legalities of refusing treatment. If he were a minor, a ward of the state or a dependant, his case would not have been so straightforward. But he is a cognitively intact 78-year-old man and he has full say over his treatment.

'No, no.' I remind myself that I can quibble with him over the substance but not the morality of his decision.

He is enigmatic. On the one hand, he seems well-spoken, world-wise and likeable. He seems to care for his wife and son, for whom he has an obvious tender spot. But on the other hand, he does not seem to concern himself too deeply with their ongoing welfare, for he must surely realise the toll his premature death will exact on his vulnerable family. The more I see him, the more the questions eat at me. What sort of a person would do this? What right does he have to use me as a care provider but only for the care he wants? Can I refuse to see him because I find his behaviour objectionable? But, I remind myself, he behaves appropriately and respectfully towards me, it is just that I don't agree with his decision. And anyway, what right do I have to act as his moral compass?

I discuss his case with a colleague. 'That's sad,' he says. 'But it's his choice.'

'I know, but haven't you had instances where you can't reconcile with a patient's choice?'

He passes his hand over his head in a flying motion. 'That's when you have to let it go.'

I know he is right but I can't shake off the feeling that I need to advocate for the needs of his family, who probably do not even know the extent of his condition. But the weeks continue to slip by without resolution.

The next time, he looks worse. He is pale and in more pain. He takes a tablet out of his pocket and tucks it into the corner of his mouth before taking a swig of coffee. 'This will give me enough time, if you keep it short.' We both smile.

'How are you doing?' he starts off.

'Better if you skip the traffic report!' I say with a mock plea.

'I have done them all, I suspect! Doc, I feel terrible.'

I listen to the list of his symptoms and examine him.

'There is fluid in your lungs. Have you been short of breath?'

'Yeah, I can't chase my son around anymore. I know it's spreading.'

A scan proves him correct.

'I knew it.' I watch him carefully for any signs of remorse but he says this more as a statement of fact.

'We can make your breathing easier by removing some of the fluid.'

'No, it's okay.'

'It doesn't take long and only needs a local anaesthetic.'

'No, I will put up with it.'

I raise my eyebrows. 'It could get troublesome.'

'We will see.'

'Do you want me to adjust your painkillers?'

'Yes, maybe.'

'You could be anaemic. Would you like me to check your bloods?'

'Not today.'

I am exasperated. I feel as if he is intentionally making me work against my grain. My natural instinct as his doctor is to want to help him, make him feel better, if not live longer. Otherwise what is the sense in listening to his compendium of symptoms that he could recite to a stranger at the bus stop?

'Okay,' I reply. 'Let me know when you want some help.'

'Are you annoyed, doctor?'

'Actually, I feel like I can't do anything right by you.'

'Why?'

'Why?' I look at him incredulously. Surely he is playing me for a fool.

'Oh, because I didn't take your initial advice about removing the kidney?'

I decide that contrary to his initial instructions, he is willing to have a longer conversation.

'The kidney cancer which has now spread.'

He ignores the implied accusation in my voice and says, 'Don't you have other patients who don't follow your recommendation?'

Yes, but they tend not to be the ones who have a young wife and child, I want to retort, but bite my tongue.

'Every now and then.'

'So I am one of them.'

'You know it's not as simple as that, but we don't have to talk about it.' I decide that as my colleague suggested, I really will let it go. His wife and son are not my patients. I have met them once, don't know about their circumstances and have enough issues to focus on without adding imagined ones to the list. But this meeting has awoken within him a desire to talk and convince me of his side of the story.

'You think I am selfish, don't you?'

I don't reply.

'I am seventy-nine next month. Tell me, at what point does a man become entitled to think of himself alone? You say the surgery is simple, but you don't know that. What if I became disabled afterwards? At my age, it would be straight to a nursing home. How long would I have to live like that? Two years, three, five? With a nonexistent quality of life. How would my wife cope with the enormous strain? What would be my son's memory of me?'

'Who will look after your wife and son once you die?'

'They will look after each other without interference from a dependent old husband and father. You say that the surgery could potentially cure me, but there is a chance that the cancer would return. In this life, nothing is assured. I weighed up my chances and didn't like mine.'

'But is your wife even aware of this reasoning or does she think I am not treating you?'

'She grew up in a poor village where she was surrounded by death. She can smell death. Before you wonder, she doesn't know that I could have had surgery and I don't think it would be fair to ask her to be involved in that decision. She would simply have said it was up to me. And if she secretly wanted me to have the surgery and I didn't, she would have felt more hurt.'

'I feel concerned for your family. Your wife seems so vulnerable.'

'But there comes a point in life when an individual must take responsibility for oneself. My wife is well provided for. It will be hard but she knew when she married me that I would die before her. She knew that I would not see our son grow up but she wanted to have a child to accompany her in her own life. I bet society would consider this merely fulfilling a maternal longing. I am not selfish but I'm doing what's right for me. I suspect you frequently say this to your patients.'

There is cogency and a refreshing honesty within his explanation and it makes me feel less certain about having judged him. He is right that all too often, medicine promises more than it can deliver and what may be broadly true about his disease may not apply to his individual case.

'I am glad you told me how you feel. I think it clears up some things for me,' I offer.

'In my life I have done many different jobs and met many people. And I have learnt that people generally have a good reason for doing what they do. The challenge is in understanding their motive before judging them.' I feel duly chastised.

His appearances at clinic slowly drop away as he tries to conserve his energy and deal with his symptoms. At my repeated urging, he reluctantly accepts help from the palliative care nurses, whose ongoing involvement he then embraces. His wife continues to devote her energies to him and, remarkably, arranges with his friend to take the family away for a weekend at his favourite beach. He tells me that it was one of the best times he had ever spent with his son. 'We say it all the time but I know now that every moment truly was precious and irreplaceable.'

The last time I see him he looks so frail that I know there will be no further conversations.

'You know the offer for hospice is still open.'

'I will think about it.'

His wife looks on quietly as his weight rests on her tiny frame.

I adjust his pain medications, prescribe him sleeping tablets for his increasingly disrupted sleep, and see him off in a wheelchair. I give him another appointment slip out of habit and politeness, not wanting to make it any more obvious that the end is near.

When he is distracted, I slip his wife the phone number for the hospice. On it, I have written in bold letters: 'If too sick, phone for help.'

By the way in which she secretes it into the pocket of her jeans without changing her expression, I know that she is not as naive as I have made her out to be. And in spite of having thought that I had made peace with his decision, I feel my uncertainty return. Why didn't she say something? Was it because she thought I was his advocate and not hers? Did she fight with him over his decision to die? Does she feel I colluded with him?

The very next week, his palliative care nurse sends me a note to say he died but in the rush of patients, I don't ask for any other details. I resolve to call his wife but feel awkward as I never really knew her.

Many months later, the story comes full circle in an astonishing way. I am conducting job interviews for junior doctors. It is late in the afternoon and it is becoming harder to sustain the panel's attention.

'Tell us about a difficult situation that you have encountered and what you learnt from it,' my associate's voice drones over the stale air in the room. After three hours of repeating the same questions, we can hear each other think the same thought: 'Please let it be interesting, something other than a conflict with a bossy nurse or your lazy intern.'

The trainee seated before us actually pauses to consider her answer. I already feel encouraged. She thinks some more and from her expression, it is clear that she is making a split-second decision. My colleague taps a pencil distractedly, causing her to jump slightly.

'I am not sure if this counts,' she begins, 'but during my palliative care rotation, I took care of an old man who was dying of metastatic renal cell cancer. He came in very unwell. While admitting him, I discovered that he had refused treatment for the initial cancer, which was thought to be curable. I thought that was interesting but when I met his young wife and five-year-old son, I was shocked at his decision. They were so upset at his condition and kept crying. I felt really sad for their loss.'

I am entranced. It seems eerie to hear her recount her version of the story. I sit up in my chair.

'We gave him a bit of fluid that didn't really do anything, but I remember thinking that, for a time, he held this important decision in his hands. I mean, I don't know, but I felt that his son was so innocent in all of this and he was going to be without a father. I don't have any children but I couldn't imagine not doing everything you could to be with your child.'

Visibly moved by the memory, she stops to collect herself. The interviewer next to me tenses in her chair. I feel an unwelcome and completely unexpected sense of deja vu.

She tries to shrug dismissively but the gesture fails. 'I felt conflicted looking after this man but didn't really have a choice. When he died a few days later, I felt relieved in a way because I wouldn't have to see his family again but also guilty that I was judging him.'

She looks at us and stops self-consciously, thinking she has crossed the line. She hastily and mildly concludes, 'I guess what I learnt from this experience was that you have to learn to respect the patient's wishes even if you don't agree, but I still think about the case.'

In front of her, I feel burdened by my secret. She obviously has not connected the patient with his oncologist. In a hospital that serves thousands of cancer patients, my colleague also has no reason to. But she is clearly touched by the story and by the impression it left on the candidate. At the end of the interview, she says, 'Maybe you should try to talk to the patient's oncologist. It might help you make sense of what happened.'

She looks at her gratefully. 'I've thought about it but feel foolish. I don't remember the exact wording but the letters suggested that the oncologist was quite comfortable with his decision.'

I wonder if she can sense my silent dissent.

And then the candidate's final candid observation, perhaps made to console herself: 'I guess this is why it takes so many years to become a specialist – you have to learn how to separate your feelings from the facts. I am sure it was just me.'

'You'd be surprised,' I reply in my mind.

We politely shake her hand and wish her good luck. The door closes behind her.

'Well!' my colleague says, turning to me. 'What do you think of that?'

'You first,' I urge.

15

◇

You have such grace

In the motley crowd that lines the seats of the waiting room, he cuts an unusual figure. Patients shuffle in narrow, uncomfortable chairs, looking up eagerly as a doctor emerges from one of the many offices and stands facing the room. Eyes firmly fixed on the file, the doctor calls out a name. A hand shoots up followed by 'I am here, I am here.' An elderly lady slowly makes her way towards the doctor, carefully navigating her wheeled frame to avoid the feet, coats and X-ray envelopes that line her path. Their short-lived anticipation blotted out again, the remaining patients go back to marking time before another doctor comes out.

Someone picks up a tattered crossword puzzle torn from the end of a magazine and resumes where another bored patient left off. Another shakes his head and jabs at his phone, probably sending a message that the doctors are running late again. A few patients simply sink back exhaustedly into their seat, veterans of a game where the allocated and real appointment times differ by the customary one hour. But as I usher patients in and out of my own office, I keep noticing a man near the front of the waiting room. He is dressed in a smart navy jacket paired with beige trousers, supporting a slim briefcase on his knees. His thick brown hair is neatly combed to remove all but the slightest suggestion of a wave. He sits calmly but alertly, ready to leap at the first summons. But his expression is not one of apprehension or uneasiness but rather, mirrors his posture. It is as if he has dropped into this room full of oncology patients to record his observations.

The afternoon wears on but the waiting room seems no less full. I rub my forehead, hoping to erase the beginnings of a headache. I look down at his file to avoid the countless pairs of eyes that hope to be next.

'Mr Tom Cleary,' I announce.

He approaches me eagerly. I hold the door open for him but he steps aside, allowing me to enter first. I sit down and direct him to a chair.

'Is there anyone else coming in?'

'No, no. I am alone.'

'Mr Cleary,' I say after the initial introduction, 'my job today is to ask you a series of questions, examine you and talk to you about the diagnosis and what we do from here. Please bear with me as I do the initial talking. I will give you plenty of time to ask me questions along the way.'

'Sure. Please call me Tom.'

Tom is a youthful 58-year-old who has never been sick in his life. Recently, he happened to play in a local squash competition and met his family doctor on the opposing team. Later she observed that he looked pale and had become unusually short of breath during play. She asked him to see her the next day and when he did, a chest X-ray revealed a suspicious mass in the lung. A biopsy confirmed malignant cells. After organising some urgent tests, she has sent him to the oncology clinic.

'Tom, I am afraid the tests show that you have lung cancer.'

'Yes, my doctor told me as much.'

'Did she say anything else?'

'No, she said it was best to get all the information on it from an oncologist.'

I discuss the diagnosis in some detail. 'I never smoked, never drank,' he says. I tell him that in a minority of cases, non-smokers too can be afflicted with the disease. He leans forward and nods as if absorbing a lecture. His entire being looks interested; I note that he is not frightened or shaken by the revelation, obviously having had the time to digest the initial shock.

'Your CT suggests that the cancer is localised to the right lung. In that case, it is possible that it can be removed via operation.'

'Okay, so what do we do? Where do I see a surgeon?'

'First we need another scan that allows us to see if the disease is truly localised, or whether there are other spots invisible on a CT.'

For the first time his face falls. 'You mean a CT can lie?'

'Not lie so much as be limited in its ability to detect very small spots.'

He promptly agrees to the additional tests. While I fill out the forms, we talk about what is loosely termed 'social history', its bland name belying the vital pieces of information it contains about the patient as a person.

'Are you married?' I ask.

'Yes. No. Well, not anymore. But it was an amicable separation,' he quickly adds with a reassuring smile.

'Any children?'

'One beautiful daughter, seventeen.'

'What did you use to do?'

'Use to? I still do! I run my own photography business. It's grown immensely and I am a little concerned about how much time off this will need. For example, if I have an operation for the cancer, how long will the recovery take?'

'Let's wait and see what the new scan shows.' As I make a review appointment, I hope that I have some good news to deliver to this affable man.

It is not to be. The new scan lights up with black spots in a number of bones. My heart sinks as he regards me with anticipation.

'Tom, I am sorry to say that the cancer has spread beyond the lung into the bones, mostly the ribs.'

He is crestfallen. 'You know, I have ignored the pain in my chest for months, thinking it was the strain from squash.'

The rest of our conversation takes on a more sombre tone than either of us wishes. The intent of treatment suddenly changed from curative to palliative, I talk to Tom about having chemotherapy in an effort to delay the progression of the disease and the onset of new symptoms. I tell him that although I cannot rid him of his cancer, there are many medications and technology to keep him comfortable and pain-free.

His expression relaxes. 'Thank you, that's what I needed to hear.'

After some time, I say, 'Is there anything else you want to ask me?'

Although I have tried to be thorough, I would have thought that a man so used to being in control would ply me with count-less questions, wanting to know all the details. But, standing up, he shakes my hand and says, 'I feel that you have given me a very good idea of what to expect. I am sure there will be questions later but not right now.'

I have just told a man absorbed in his life and profession that he has not long to live. No matter how many times I deliver this news, my heart still feels wrenched in the process. I look back on my words even as I say them. Was I too plain-spoken or coy? Was I cheerless or honest? Did I leave room for a glimmer of hope in a crowd of sobering facts?

Although it is never possible to know exactly what a patient thinks of the initial conversation, I find myself calmed by Tom's tranquillity. His conduct is a welcome counterbalance to that of the afternoon's other patients, who turn out to be far more unnerved and highly strung about their cancer journey.

The initial chemotherapy produces a good response. He experiences little of the nausea or infection risk that I warn him about and his pain settles down nicely. He overcomes his fatigue well and, to his relief, is able to keep working long hours. Our conversations during chemotherapy were short and revolved mainly around tackling side effects, but now, at the end of the prescribed course of treatment, we sit down to discuss the future.

I study his scans and carefully check the report to be sure. No new disease has emerged and the primary lung cancer has shrunk to half its original size. The scan taken together with his well-being is encouraging, I say. He beams like a proud schoolboy who has completed his homework as instructed. It seems almost malevolent to remind him that, given the treacherous disease that lung cancer is, his response is going to be tentative and his relief only good until the next clinic appointment. I take a slightly different approach.

'Tom, we will have to keep a very close eye on you as there is still potential for you to experience trouble. I will need to see you every month and we will have to do tests from time to time.'

'Of course, I understand that this is a bad disease and I am not immune from it. But it's great that you are going to keep an eye on me. I already feel better knowing that I have somewhere to come back to!'

I can't help but smile at a patient who thinks the world of his doctor for making a follow-up appointment. If only all patients were so easily pleased. Tom would be a natural case study for the role of positive thinking in cancer outcomes. Then, shortly before I am due to see him again, I have to go on emergency leave during my pregnancy and must cancel my appointments at short notice. I wonder about him and other patients but, confined to bed and soon preoccupied with my own troubles, I reluctantly cede my duties to colleagues.

When I return a few months after giving birth, I have lost track of several patients. Unfortunately, a gap of only a few months has translated into the death of a substantial number; I remind myself to call families when I have settled back into the rhythm of things. Like many in public hospitals, patients here are not assigned to an individual oncologist but must wait in queue to see the next available doctor. The ethos is that the mix of the new and old patients, with a variety of conditions, contributes to trainee education and allows more than one oncologist to guide the treatment. In theory, the model ought to foster partnership, discussion and intellectual drive; however, for many patients the practice is unsatisfactory, and sometimes distressing. When a patient is seen by three different oncologists in as many appointments, the common perception is that no single individual is responsible for the patient's management. Occasionally we get around the problem by keeping an eye out for patients we know well, but this is adhoc and unreliable at the best of times.

Then I run into Tom in the waiting room. My look of surprise at simply seeing him alive is matched by his pleasure at seeing a familiar face again. I usher him into my room followed by his exclamations of delight.

'You simply disappeared one day,' he said.

'I am sorry, it was quite sudden,' I reply.

'But one of the best reasons in the world to disappear from work!' Before I can read more into his statement, he offers, 'Congratulations on the birth of your little girl!' I am touched by his attention to detail.

A woman follows him into the room with a smile. She gently holds him by the arm as he seats himself.

'This is my wife, Ivana.'

I am sure he said he was separated but they seem at ease with each other. I wonder whether his disease has brought them back together. She is pleasant, informed and not afraid to contradict him.

He brings me up to date in his customary concise and measured way. 'After I saw you and you said things looked good, I went back to playing squash. I was doing well and then I became short of breath again. I knew something was wrong. It turned out that my lung was full of fluid. Another oncologist sent me for an operation and they got three litres out. I have never felt the same since.'

His face is thinner and his ribs more prominent. Although there is no one particularly noticeable abnormality, his previous vitality seems replaced by a general languor, rendered all the more evident to me because of the gap between our consultations. I know the look well – the insidious creep of cancer on the unsuspecting patient.

'You feel terrible,' Ivana chips in. 'You are uncomfortable breathing, your pain is worse, and you are just not right.'

He nods self-consciously, reluctant to be a nuisance.

'Have you had a scan lately?'

'I am supposed to but just haven't felt well enough,' he confesses, relieved to have the matter out in the open.

'Get it on a Tuesday as I don't teach any classes then,' Ivana suggests. She goes out to book the appointment before he changes his mind.

'How are you managing at home?' I ask, concerned about whether he is alone.

'Ivana and my daughter are there, it's been fine. You know this is the first time in years that we have had so much time at home. It makes you wonder about all that wasted time.'

Even behind closed doors, his reference to the marriage is so courteous that I am led to wonder whether the separation was in his mind only and something that he has now put behind him. She has not alluded to it and, the way she behaves, I wonder if she even knew what was on his mind. I leave the matter alone, satisfied that he is being well looked after.

Tom's new scans explain the reason for his deterioration. The cancer has spread.

'I knew it,' he says, making a wry face. 'You always said it would come back.'

I wait for him to ask about having more therapy; instead, he adjusts himself in his chair, leans forward and says, 'I have a number of things that I need to take care of before I die. I would appreciate it if we could have a frank discussion about my condition and what is going to happen to me.' As if to reassure me, he says, 'I am not scared to die but I need to know how it will happen.'

I let go of my pen, poised on the consent form for chemotherapy. One would expect these conversations to be a routine part of being an oncologist but it is surprising how many patients choose not to know the details around their decline and eventual death. It is understandable in other ways – doctors are not good at predicting life spans and many do not feel equipped to handle such conversations, which are admittedly fraught with uncertainty and uncomfortable to engage in. For many patients, every interaction with their doctor already seems profound and the future already grim without additional details.

'What do you want to know, Tom? I will try to be frank.'

He looks at his wife before continuing. 'I thought it would be easier if I made a list – I have been writing these questions for the last few days.' He hands over the list. On it, in neat and precise writing, I read the following questions:

How will I die?

Will it be sudden?

Can you keep me out of pain?

Can I go away on holiday?

How many more decent days are there left?

Despite my training, I am taken aback by the questions. They strike right at the core of the fears of most patients but it needs Tom's mettle to put them into words. Filled with respect for his dignified conduct, I set about to address the points. I go back to pretending I am in an exam, where two sets of expectations have to be addressed – the patient's need for truth and sensitivity and the examiner's for accuracy of detail. It can be tricky to balance both. I take pains to stipulate that this is only my opinion. Nevertheless, I feel wretched in putting my so far nebulous private fears into such an explicit message. What if I am wrong, I wonder. What if Tom is the one to defy predictions and one day prove the subject of discussion and debate? What if he is still sitting at the front of the waiting room a few years hence pointing at me as the doctor who gave him only months to live? I know that every oncologist has an anecdote like this – and although the patient feels only joy and relief at having beaten the odds, the doctor is left to toy with doubts over how he could have got things so wrong. But Tom's keen and attentive questions gradually assure me that he is more likely to reproach me for withholding my thoughts than for getting some of the details wrong.

When I finally stop talking, I feel as if I have gone on for far longer than invited. But Tom repays me with his hallmark spirited answer.

'That's great! Thank you. After that talk, I feel like I have a plan and that's all I can ask you for.'

I look on in amazement as he says, 'I am going to hold off on more treatment which could give me nasty side effects and take my wife and daughter on a holiday. I am going to keep my business open but wind it down and leave it in good order.'

'You need better pain relief if you are going away,' the practical Ivana reminds him. I study her expression but she seems to be equally at peace with her husband's decision. Thus reminded, Tom winces.

I prescribe him a small dose of morphine and warn him about the usual side effects. Writing out the prescription, I ask the usual question: 'Is there anything else?'

They look at each other. 'Can I see you when I come back? It's so much easier talking to someone who knows me.'

The problem of not having an assigned oncologist becomes especially relevant when a patient begins a sensitive discussion with one doctor and establishes a rapport, only to find himself having to start all over again when his file is picked up by someone else. I am conscious that it has taken Tom tremendous emotional investment to arrive at his list of questions and am keen to spare him additional effort.

Breaking with tradition, I hand him a note, specifying that he should see me on his repeat appointments. It seems unfair to the rest of the patients who do not receive this additional advocacy but I feel unable to deny Tom's reasonable request. I make a mental note to remind the secretary.

'I am really grateful to you for all the trouble you are taking.'

It is amazing how a sincere thank you can transform the spirit of a day.

'Tom, you have such grace,' I marvel as I see him out. He beams.

Tom returns two weeks later than anticipated for his next review. He extended his holiday at the beach because he felt so relaxed. However, he tells me that the last few days have again seen a sharp decline in his comfort. He is running out of breath in the shower and his pain has become more persistent. New areas of pain have developed, his back being particularly bothersome. I increase his painkillers, arrange for radiation therapy to his painful bones, and start him on different chemotherapy drugs with his permission.

He huddles in his chair, breathing shallow breaths with effort.

'It's this damned breathing,' he sighs. 'If only I could fill my lungs with air, I would feel so much better. But I feel as if someone is squashing my chest and I just can't fill up.' If a medical student were with me, I would tell her that this is an apt description of air hunger. He declines my offer to admit him to hospital. 'No, if the end is coming, I want to be home.' However, he eagerly accepts home oxygen.

He is back within two weeks with an angry rash on his face and body as a result of the chemotherapy. The softest clothes hurt when they brush against his peeling skin. He looks wasted. My heart sinks. I take his hand carefully to ease him into the chair. His skin feels alien, like sandpaper. When he gets his breath back and notices my dismay at his disfigured face, he quips, 'Thank God I don't have to go to the prom any time soon, huh?'

Despite his obvious discomfort, I laugh aloud at the thought. His wife and he join in. Our laughter serves to defuse the tension. I am sure he planned it that way and feel grateful.

'Let's not discuss this drug at all,' he says, 'because whether it's working or not, I have had enough.'

I let him take the lead. 'What would you like me to do, Tom?'

'Tell me that it's okay to stop treatment.'

'It is.'

'I feel worse. Can you tell me how long I could have now?'

I have never become used to his dispassionate style of discussing his own life expectancy.

'Tom, I agree you do look worse.'

'Are we talking days, weeks?'

'It could be either, probably the latter.'

'Okay.'

'What can I do for you?' I tell myself all my words will sound equally hollow.

'I don't think you can do anything, doctor.'

'The palliative care team may need to increase their visits.' I introduced him to the nurses several months ago but he hasn't needed them so far.

'Does he have enough prescriptions?' I ask Ivana.

'Yes, to last him into the next world, he complains!'

He shakes his head. 'It's amazing how many different medications I have needed just in the last few months. How do people cope with such complex stuff? Most days, I feel too tired to even read the names of my pills. If it were not for my family, I would simply not take them. They should get some credit, you know.' I nod in appreciation of another perceptive comment from this extraordinary man.

Having exhausted treatment and conversation, I suddenly realise that this may be the last time I see Tom. I feel sad at the impending loss of his company after more than a year of regular visits that I looked forward to. I chastise myself that this is an object lesson in the need to keep patients at arm's length, but who could fail to be inspired by Tom's indomitable spirit and gracious manners?

'Tom,' I ask slowly, 'you probably don't need to drag yourself in here again for an appointment with me, but do you want one anyway?'

I am sure he will read into this my final goodbye but instead he jumps at the offer.

'Yes please! I would feel better knowing that I am booked in.'

'Sure.'

'It's funny,' he explains, 'but when you have cancer, other doctors don't want to touch you for fear of upsetting something.'

He doesn't have to explain why he wants to come back. I find myself curiously relieved that I don't have to take my leave yet.

Four weeks pass and when I don't see Tom in clinic, I assume that he has died. I ask the secretary to call for his file so I can check on his wife. Then, walking out of my room to see another patient, I see Tom and Ivana slowly walking ahead of me.

'Tom!' I can't contain my surprise at finding him in clinic.

He turns around slowly, leaning heavily against his wife, out of breath and words. I feel an instant of dread in my heart. Since I specified it, I have been the only doctor Tom has seen in clinic for the last several months. Did he change his mind and come to see someone else, in which case, should I interfere? It is too late to think about it now as he walks towards me.

'Come in,' I urge. 'I was going to call you today!' I omit to mention that I was not expecting him to answer the phone.

Ivana shuts the door behind them.

'How are you?' I ask.

Tom, a paragon of stoicism until now, bursts into tears. I watch in utter amazement. My first selfish thought is that whoever he just saw has just told him I got it wrong.

As his tears keep falling, Ivana says, 'The clerk said I couldn't insist on seeing you if you were busy because this is a public clinic. So we saw another doctor. He said there was nothing else to offer

Tom.' It is her turn to cry. Although I am irritated by the clerk's well-meant but insensitive approach, I am more puzzled by their response to something that I have discussed with them on many occasions.

Tom wipes his eyes and waves a slip. 'And because there is nothing else, he wrote "No further appointment."' He continues haltingly, 'This is the only place and you are the only doctor I have known since I was diagnosed. I know I don't strictly need you but to tell the truth, I feel abandoned.'

I stare at Tom. He is trembling. In all the time that I have known him, from the initial surprise of his diagnosis through the later challenges, he has never looked as rattled, as vulnerable as now. Could this complete change in his behaviour really be due to a meaningful attachment that has grown over time?

I am overwhelmed by remorse. In a desperate bid to erase Tom's hurt, I say, 'Well, that may be true, but I would really like to see you again, so would you come back to let me know how you are doing?'

Out of the corner of my eye, I see Ivana's shoulders relax.

Tom grips the handles of his chair. 'Really?'

'Yes, I like seeing you, Tom.'

'You don't mind? I mean, it won't waste your time?'

My heart melts at his childlike plea. 'I *like* seeing you, Tom,' I repeat for effect.

Taking the appointment slip in my hand, I ask, 'Shall we make it one week or two?' I fear that anything else would be too long.

'Two weeks would be fine, thank you.'

'Tom, I will personally look out for you in the waiting room and get you.'

Relief floods his face. I can only think how narrowly and serendipitously I avoided consigning Tom to a final state of despair.

Tom spontaneously hugs me and says, 'This is the single most useful visit I have had. Thank you for standing by me.'

I have heard many dramatic pronouncements from patients but this one is compelling, for it makes me realise that the things doctors don't think twice about sometimes matter the most to patients. Like the doctor who saw Tom, I too discharge patients from clinic, either because they are stable or because they don't need active treatment by an oncologist. Now I have seen for myself that the decision is not so straightforward and patients can experience a traumatic separation from their doctor.

Exactly one week later, I receive a phone call from his wife. 'Tom passed away last night,' she tells me.

Despite anticipating this, I feel a rush of regret at the news. 'I am very sorry. Was he comfortable?'

'You won't believe this. We had dinner in the garden last night with some of his best friends. He had a great time. They left and he came inside to get changed for bed. He was sitting on the edge of the bed and telling me how happy he was and then he just fell backwards. His heart had stopped.'

We talk some more. She is sad but clearly relieved that the ordeal has ended for them all. We reminisce a little about Tom. Her impressions of him from their heady days together are different from mine, gathered when he was at his lowest. But on one thing we agree – Tom himself could not have scripted a better end to a quietly remarkable life.

16

◇

It's hard to let go

'Is there any money we need to pay? Is that why you won't treat him?'

I know her only as Isobel. Her face wears a hunted expression, her slender frame weighed down by fatigue and untold distress. In her native country people died for lack of sufficient funds to afford treatment. It was one of the reasons she and her husband left their poverty-stricken life and, along with it, their extensive clan. They saw her mother die of pneumonia, a disease the village elders who could read said was treatable in foreign countries. And that was another thing. They wanted their children to be educated, like those few village elders, and not to become mere peasants who spent their lives at the mercy of a landowner. Saying goodbye seemed easier when they thought of the twin boons of free health care and education.

'No, no,' I hurry to reassure her. 'This has nothing to do with money. It is just that he is not well enough to have treatment.'

'Anything, doctor; we will do anything to make him better. We have three young children.' She unconsciously fingers the gold chain around her neck.

'I know . . .'

She walks down the corridor, whispering a prayer. I feel sick with the unfairness of life.

He felt well two months ago. Last month, he developed an irritating cough that would not go away. A CT scan of his chest revealed suspicious lumps. Before the family doctor could figure out where to send him, he fainted from anaemia. It was only after he had had time to think that he remembered he had been experiencing a lot of heartburn lately. He did not understand why one doctor said to another, 'There is the culprit!' After all, everyone got heartburn from time to time – wasn't it a sign of his wife's sumptuous cooking?

A gastroscopy uncovered a sinister gastric cancer. Simultaneously his liver function started to deteriorate. His doctors requested an oncology consultation.

I first met the patient and his wife on the medical unit on a consult. He walked in slowly from the bathroom, his arm stabilising a tottering IV pole with a saline bag on top. His skin was jaundiced, his face filled with the tell-tale signs of sleepless nights. Small pieces of cotton wool marked failed attempts to find a vein.

'He has lost a lot of weight and his back hurts,' his wife offered.

'I am tired and sweating a lot,' he added.

I was not surprised at the revelation. His cancer looked aggressive. His physiological reserve was dissipating every day and he had already required three bags of blood. The skyrocketing liver function readings beggared belief. The diagnosis of advanced cancer had been clearly established but for an unexpected occurrence – repeated X-rays failed to demonstrate any distinct liver abnormality even as the liver continued to fail. What one would commonly expect to see in this situation is a liver crowded with metastases, the lesions suffocating normal tissue, sabotaging normal function.

Unexpected and not easily explainable findings in patients lead to academic curiosity, and thus it was in his case. What was causing the man's liver to fail? Was it the cancer, and if so, why was it invisible? Or had the prolonged use of multiple antibiotics for a presumed chest infection led to the disaster? Or did he harbour another, yet undiagnosed disease? Experts were summoned to the bedside but with the numbers worsening faster than one could carry out blood tests, the question posed more interest than immediate relevance.

Sitting at the foot of the bed, I advised the couple of the seriousness of his situation and the limitation in offering chemotherapy due to his failing liver and blood counts. They absorbed some of the news but their chief concern was that he be transferred to the oncology unit where treatment could start urgently. They did not feel that the current team understood his parlous state or was capable of managing his further care. I did not think he would recover enough to receive chemotherapy but hoped that the oncology unit was better equipped to deal with the many ramifications of the tragic situation unfolding before us.

'So is there nothing you can do to cure Carlos?' his wife simultaneously asked and pleaded. I had strived to curb the impulsive stream of false reassurances about to spring from my lips and corrected her gently.

'There may not be any chemotherapy we can give but there are other things we can do to make him more comfortable.'

While the weary patient looked longingly towards the exit, Isobel was unconvinced. She did not believe that an oncology consult conducted on a different ward carried the same significance as advice dispensed on an oncology unit.

'Maybe when he gets to oncology, they will think of something else,' she murmured to no one in particular. My heart felt heavy.

I prayed that in exchange for her unshakable belief, the oncology unit would offer him more than a change of scenery.

He has now been on the oncology ward for three days. Daily blood tests define a dismal trail, his hemoglobin and bilirubin edging dangerously towards the wrong ends of the spectrum. Having handed over his day-to-day management to the team based on the oncology ward, I drop by to see him. The IV pole is still attached to his arm. A card hung by his bed advises he now needs one-person assistance to walk. A tray of food remains untouched, the menu for the next meal unfilled. The jaundice penetrates every pore of his skeletal body. He looks eerie.

'They are waiting to see what the liver does,' Isobel relays. 'He could still have some treatment . . .' She fingers the cross on her gold chain.

Out of the corner of my eye, I see Carlos look less hopeful, and ask, 'Have you thought of getting home for a while? Maybe a few hours outside will feel good.' A cold and rainy winter has finally given way to the bliss of spring. The bare branches are populated with hopeful buds, there are signs of green wherever the eye looks, and the sun, once again, has returned with heartening warmth. The outside looks good even through perspex. I yearn for him to feel it again. It would make him feel better than anything being done indoors.

His face breaks into a smile. With childlike eagerness, he says, 'I have a strong faith. I believe in God. It would be so good to get to church on Sunday. Maybe I could get home for a few hours.'

What would he ask his God? For there to be a miraculous cure or salvation from suffering? To give his wife the courage to take him home or the strength to deal with his loss?

'I am sure that going to church would be fine.' Finally, to accede to a patient's wish.

She speaks slowly: 'But they still have to do tests . . . He can have chemo if the liver gets better.'

'They will do nothing new on Sunday,' I say soothingly. I know them, I work with them. I know what *they* know. I try to keep it simple for her. 'His liver has a long way to go before he would be safe to have chemotherapy. Going to church might take his mind off things.'

Perhaps she thinks the path he would take is from church straight to home. Perhaps she cannot believe that a test on Sunday won't provide the answer they are looking for.

'No one else suggested going out.' She says it too quickly for me to separate accusation from fact. His eyes look out wistfully.

That doesn't mean I am wrong, I want to plead with him. When you are in hospital, our primary responsibility is to treat you, to order tests and drugs, to finesse the ways in which we can fix your broken body. But now that we have sold you such hope, we become so wedded to our ideals that we shy away from reality. The truth is we cannot deliver. The truth is you are dying and no one quite knows how or when to tell you. The tests are a proxy of our failed courage. I have made this mistake many times and am trying to avoid it now. Not being the primary oncologist involved in your day-to-day care also gives me some objectivity, which is difficult to come by in testing circumstances like yours.

But I only say, 'I am sure the ward doctors would permit you to go to church.'

Her expression is firm and his desire soon dissipates, hostage to a futile hope of therapy fuelled by his wife's desperation. He mentions the confusion surrounding medical conversations and expresses a desire to 'know for sure'. Other statements from him and his wife indicate that they have sized up the ominous nature of his disease quite adequately. He knows he is dying. We know he is dying. But it is the elephant in the room we are reluctant to acknowledge while we find ourselves distractions that will carry us into another day.

Sunday passes and he does not make it to church. Monday and Tuesday also come and go, and so into another week. He undergoes an astounding array of tests and fields multiple questions, expecting a turnaround any day now even as he presides over the decline of his body. First the walls confine him, then the limitations of his physicians. We sidestep the conversation about prognosis, so much more at ease with nominating the various reasons his liver could be failing, and with ordering new tests whose only value lies in permitting us to avoid a meaningful discussion about palliation. Each time he edges towards closure, our conversations imply new and confusing avenues of hope, to carry over to the next ward round. We may not do this intentionally but it is easier than facing what stares us in the eye. I curse modern medicine that innocently permits us such an excuse.

His failing liver has stained his skin with a deep, striking yellow, against which the gleaming white of his teeth looks macabre. His dim, hollow eyes, bloated abdomen and lax skin folds add to the confronting image. The oncology trainee catches me completely by surprise when he reveals that a liver biopsy is being contemplated. He explains that they may give him 'a bit of chemo' afterwards. I stop mid-step, staring at him in amazement.

'He is desperate; he will take anything for his children.'

'Even an early, toxicity-driven death?' I ask, dismayed at our inability to recognise our own limitations.

'But he is so young,' the fellow protests. 'It's hard to let go.'

'Have you tried?'

'It's not really an experiment I feel up to. And it's not something I see other oncologists wanting to do.'

'He signed the consent form for a liver biopsy?' I ask, still reeling in disbelief.

'Yes.'

'What did you tell him?' I can't help asking before I catch myself. 'I am sorry. You know him well and I am sure you went through all the usual risks.'

'I guess we are not really sure if it will change anything either.'

We part ways, my mind screaming with frustration. I realise he has hit the nail on the head. It *is* hard to let go. There is little room in our psyche for accepting the wrath of nature or the vagaries of the human constitution. It is hard to let go and no one really teaches us how. It is surely not the first time that an unnecessary test is being performed on a patient. But given the circumstances, this one seems particularly intrusive and, to my judgement, ethically questionable. But I hurry to remind myself that my own judgement has often been fallible and perhaps it is nothing more than my overly fatalistic attitude that needs correcting. Patients come in all forms and so do their doctors. It is time for me to leave this patient in the hands of those who know him best.

I find Carlos lying in bed, his wife pacing the corridor.

'I can't believe this', she says, her tear-streaked face a heart-rending sight.

'What do you mean?'

'He is looking so bad. I came here with much hope but I think he has got worse every single day. The tests have done no good.'

I ask him how he feels.

'Not so good,' he reports.

'They are having a hard time getting blood from me,' he says. I note the gentle reprimand in his voice.

'I will see that they cut back,' I promise.

'I am praying. That's the only thing that can help now.'

Muted by a rising tide of sadness, all I can muster is, 'Prayer can be very helpful in such times.' I think cynically that prayer has a greater chance of benefiting him than chemotherapy. Many patients have said that prayer infuses some spirituality and meaning into tragic situations. If we cannot ease him into his situation, we ought to be grateful for his trying.

He is saved from a liver biopsy by the radiologist refusing to perform it, stating that the risk of significant bleeding was too high. As if to underline that he has had enough, the patient dies the next morning.

Engulfing the room is a stunned silence, punctuated by despairing words of incredulity that this could have happened to a family man, a man who had done no wrong. There are no words of consolation powerful enough to cut through the grief. Among the staff his death causes familiar expressions of sympathy. A few of the younger nurses are visibly shaken at the script that they didn't think would end so horribly, without warning. We are all dumbfounded, in awe of a disease that struck so swiftly. His death makes us pause for thought.

As I drive home, the trainee's words echo in my ears: 'It is hard to let go.' Simultaneously, I remember myself as a trainee, hurrying to another urgent Friday night consult. As my finger jabbed anxiously at the elevator button, my consultant remarked, 'The most difficult lesson you will learn is when to stand back and do nothing.' I hope that before he finishes his training, this trainee learns how to feel comfortable caring for our patients even when he has run out of new ideas. I hope he learns that this is not an optional extra in the making of a physician.

These are exciting times in medicine. Most days, I like what I do and I am in awe of how much more my patients do. I also keep hoping that I never lose sight of the fact that no therapeutic discovery will ever dispense with the need for good judgement, sensitive communication and the art of letting go.

17

◇

Tell me the truth

In a selfish way, I am relieved that he has outlived other atrocities to prepare him for this final one. It took tremendous courage to risk fleeing his war-torn village with a child and a pregnant wife when the Bosnian war broke out. His young family endured months in refugee camps before finally being granted asylum in Australia. Since then, Luca Vinjic maintains he has spent his one miracle over and over.

It took the family some years to find its feet amidst a new culture and a foreign language. But such was the relief of escape that all other challenges seemed small in comparison and their lives flourished again. Once things settled down, Luca's wife found a doctor and urged her husband to go and see him. Luca laughed at her, insisting that he was fine, but she was persistent. Because he needed something to pass the time at the doctor's, he brought up the heartburn that had been part of his life for as long as he could recall. But to the dismay of the busy tradesman, the appointment stretched on for far too long because the elderly doctor actually became interested in his symptom. And when he left, it was to have more tests than he had undergone in all his life. Luca pledged never to see a doctor again but was recalled the very next morning. Within two days, he had undergone a major operation to remove an aggressive, bleeding stomach cancer. He surprised everyone by bouncing back quickly, only to undergo months of punishing chemotherapy. Despite having all the recommended treatment, he was given a bleak long-term outlook, but when he passed the three-year mark, his doctors sounded optimistic. At five years, they relaxed and he took their cue. At ten years, he was pronounced a survivor, this time of a war with his own body.

Barely a month later, he began experiencing abdominal pain. He joked with his wife that he was probably suffering withdrawal symptoms after finally finishing up with tests after ten years, but again, she returned him to the doctor. His surgeon confirmed the worst. The disease had returned, and done so with a vengeance, dotted throughout his abdomen, causing his bowel loops to become matted in a dysfunctional mass. Some of the bowel had also telescoped into the oesophagus, making swallowing painful. The surgeon was very regretful; gastric cancer had such a poor prognosis that he had always drawn succour from Luca's case.

His disease is inoperable. A nasojejunal tube of plastic, inserted through his nose and fed into his small bowel to assist with feeding, worsens his pain and has to be removed. A feeding jejunostomy – created by making a surgical hole in the bowel – in a heavily cancerous abdominal cavity is considered too dangerous to attempt. He has been on intravenous fluids for days while his medical team considers its options.

This morning's conference of surgeons has conceded that it is in a quandary and asks for an oncology opinion. I am asked to see him more out of wishful thinking than necessity and the referral note reflects the intern's concern. She asks for my opinion on palliative chemotherapy but it is the plea in the last line that catches my attention. 'We are concerned about our growing inability to feed or hydrate him and would be grateful for your input.'

I walk into his room to find him nodding off. A bag of saline drips through his crooked arm. His soles extend beyond the foot of the bed.

'I am the cancer doctor. Your surgeon asked me to drop in.'

'I was expecting you,' he responds weakly.

I look around for his wife but he tells me she has stepped out for lunch. 'She is always here, the poor dear. Let her have a break.' His voice is gentle and affectionate.

I ask him how he feels. He is pale and thin, with pronounced, dark brown eyes adorning an expressive face. His spacious forehead contains many furrowed lines, as if he has needed each one to ponder the challenges life has thrown him in his fifty years. His black hair is sparse now, but he would have cut a handsome figure in his youth. His limbs are long, the movements of his fingers fluid.

'My biggest problem is pain. I can't even swallow my saliva. The doctors say, "Try to eat," but they don't listen.' His face contorts with pain.

'I can see. Does the morphine help?'

'Nothing helps, doctor.'

'That's no good,' I grimace with him.

I pick up his drug chart and feel a glimmer of hope.

'You know, you are on such a tiny dose of morphine that I am not surprised it's not doing anything. I am going to increase it and see if it works.'

'Okay. Maybe that will do the trick,' he agrees obligingly.

'You look tired. Let me check in on you tomorrow to see if things are any better.'

'Okay.'

There is a slight awkwardness to this interaction. I cannot make much of him in a few minutes and he has probably heard so many doctors suggest so many ideas that he can neither discriminate between doctors or warm to an idea.

The next afternoon, Luca is asleep but wakes up at the sound of the opening door. His wife is sitting next to him, leafing through a cookbook whose recipes promise to reinvigorate the fussiest of cancer patients.

'How are you?' I smile at them both.

'The same, doctor.'

'Did you notice a change with the higher dose of morphine?'

'A little bit, I think.'

His wife is not quite as convinced but I am ready to seize on even a grain of hope in this predicament.

'Good. Let's stick to this dose for another day and see, and please make sure you tell the nurses whenever you have pain.'

'He is in *constant* pain,' she says softly.

'If morphine doesn't do anything, I will think of something else,' I reassure her, glad for a reprieve until the next day.

Again, I sense the same awkwardness, doctor and patient going through the motions, each thinking different thoughts about the same problem. I see it often and don't deal with it as well as I should. I know that my brief is to discuss chemotherapy with him but it seems farcical to do so when he can't speak a full sentence comfortably.

The next day, Liljana jumps in to stop her husband from dispensing false hope to the doctor.

'Doctor, don't listen to him. He is too nice to tell you that he is in pain, that the morphine has done nothing for him.' Her voice is half-plea and half-admonition as he looks on sheepishly.

'Liljana, you must respect the doctor, darling! She is trying her best.'

'Sorry,' she mumbles.

'Please don't say that. I am glad that you have told me the truth because I need to think some more about this now.'

A relieved Liljana taps him on the shoulder. 'See, I told you. They can't guess what's happening to you.'

I wish Liljana was right once again but it is clear what is happening to her husband.

Without treatment for the aggressive cancer and without any food for more than one week, his subsistence on intravenous fluids is beginning to show. Even in the last few days, his face has lost some of its roundness and his exposed arms look sinewy. What's more, I think he knows full well the gravity of his situation, although his wife may not. I figure that this is as good an opportunity as any to cut to the chase.

'Your surgeons can't insert a feeding tube. They have asked about chemotherapy but I am more concerned about your nourishment.'

'What will chemotherapy do?'

'In theory, it could shrink some of the tumour burden and make you feel better.'

'I don't think it will.'

'I am concerned about your lack of feeding, Mr Vinjic,' I repeat. 'I am wondering what to do about it.'

'Basically, there is no way to feed me,' he states flatly.

I shake my head regretfully. 'I can talk to your doctors again.'

He holds up his hand in surrender. 'They have all come by and said there is nothing.'

'Maybe they can get another opinion. Surgeons are a creative lot, you know.'

Despite no oral intake for days, he projects a clear mind. Adjusting his posture in bed, he says simply, 'It seems that I will die of starvation before cancer.'

He has breathed words into my fear. I scan his face; it is calm and pensive.

'I don't want chemo and I don't mind dying but it would be nice to eat and drink.'

'I understand,' I respond sombrely, wondering how to deliver the undeliverable.

I hunt for the intern on the surgical unit. She is a foreign medical graduate from China, doing only her second rotation in this hospital.

'What do you think?' she asks eagerly. We have not spoken in the last two days.

'I think he is in a terrible situation.'

I can see her searching for the right words. 'Do you think chemotherapy will help him?'

'Chemotherapy?!' I scoff. 'At this rate, he is going to be dead by the time we get a line into him.'

To my surprise, tears start to fall from her eyes and she looks aghast. 'But oncology was his last hope,' she says in a small voice.

I know now that I have been spoiling for an argument that will make me feel better.

'No! Oncology wasn't his last hope, surgery was! If only someone could be bold enough to put a tube or a hole into this guy, at least he could eat and drink on his way to death. I can't believe anybody thought chemo was the answer!'

She stares at me, unable to understand why I am in a huff and unsure how to respond. My outburst finished, I realise immediately that my anger is not directed at her or even her bosses, but at the disease that has taken charge of a patient and defied his doctors so insolently, so easily.

My enquiries soon make it apparent that Mr Vinjic's predicament has been discussed extensively. When I return to his bedside, his wife springs from her seat. I quickly tell her that I have nothing new to offer. Her face droops but he replies sagely, 'This time it won't let me escape, but it's good of you to try.'

Involuntarily, he reaches out for one of many drinks neatly arranged on the table. One sip later, he grips his throat in pain. He spits out the drink and tries to coach the saliva into a slow swallow. I can't watch him. Her eyes are fixed on me in silent accusation.

In the next few days, I see him every day and experience much moral distress. I wish he would protest or show some anger or resentment, anything to allow an opening to defend my inaction. But he is resolutely calm. I find it hard to believe that in this modern age, when there are seemingly inexhaustible ways of achieving a given outcome, we all draw a blank at Mr Vinjic. I think wryly that on most occasions, my colleagues and I have bemoaned our profession's collective inability to say no. But today, I long for the opposite, hoping someone will agree to take up his case, giving us something to feel better about, if only temporarily.

His wife calls me one morning before I get to see him. 'Doctor, he hasn't eaten for many days. They say the IV can't stay in forever because he has no veins. I am worried.'

'I understand.'

'Then he will die!' she says, bewildered at our inability to stem her husband's inexorable decline.

'I am sorry.' There is no adequate expression to encompass my feelings.

'You must know experts. Can they help?'

'Would you like a second opinion?' I bite my tongue even as I make the offer.

'Yes! Yes! That's what we should do!'

Her enthusiasm is infectious and for a moment, I too let myself imagine that some invisible force will help her husband. She immediately embraces me as her ally in the war. I feel guilty at the thought of playing for time but I consult an eminent surgeon who I know from my resident days.

'That's tough,' he sympathises. But that's as far as he will go, hesitating to even see a patient who has now been seen by many of his colleagues. 'I don't know that there are any heroic acts to perform here,' he says, a towering presence in his navy suit and impeccable bow tie. 'The best thing is to let him die.'

I look at him quizzically and it is all I can do not to retort, 'That's usually my line.'

But after exhausting this option, I find myself persistently musing over the situation, unusual even for one faced with tragedy and death on a routine basis. Discovering my own helplessness mirrored in the patient's, I realise that I am angry at having no one to be angry at. It seems absurd that in an era when the wonders of medicine seem too many to count, we cannot fulfil an urge as primal as hunger and thirst.

'What can I do to make him eat?' his wife enquires after watching him go without food and water for another week.

'You can't,' I counsel.

'But how can he live like this?' she asks, interpreting my calmness as disinterest.

We both know the answer.

He grows weaker. His occasional excursions to the bathroom with his walking frame stop.

'It takes all my mental energy to start and then I drain myself physically getting there and back. I never thought I would request a catheter.'

One afternoon, I find him alone again. His response to my perfunctory questions about his pain, thirst and hunger are predictably gracious. But there is something unspoken: our relationship has evolved and I don't feel like his treating physician because I have never done anything therapeutic for him.

Eager to find something positive about his circumstances, I remark on how he seems at peace. 'You are a good man. This is very unfair.'

'Even good men die,' he responds quietly, revealing his own sadness. 'I have known many of them.' I wince at the reference to his wartime experience, of which he has somehow managed to make a non-issue.

'Are you afraid of dying?' Sometimes I don't know why I ask the questions I do except that they seem waiting to be asked.

'No. But I find the starvation hard.'

This is the first time that he has expressed this sentiment. It is troubling to hear him say it, but I feel as if we have finally broken ground, so I continue. 'It seems like a personal failure to me that we aren't able to help you.'

'That's the most one can ask of a doctor. That means I have been in good hands.'

I think to myself that his graciousness is as incurable as his cancer.

Breathing heavily, he drags his body up the bed. The sliding covers reveal wasted muscles, parched skin.

'I have something I must ask you. I want you to tell me how I will die.' Perhaps he catches a flicker of hesitation on my face, for he adds, 'I have asked a few doctors but no one wants to. The young Chinese doctor nearly jumped out of her skin in fright and the last surgeon just gave me a funny look and said he would send someone in, as if he had no idea. But I know you can tell me. Tell me the truth.'

Expectant eyes fill his face while I wonder what I have done to deserve his confidence in being able to illustrate these grim details. Does he think this is all I *can* do, tell him about death? Or is this a transaction of trust? Although I am initially disinclined to dwell openly on his death, I also feel relieved to do something within my capacity.

He starts talking before I change my mind. Although his father ran his way out of the war, he later died of respiratory failure. Watching him gulping for air in an under-serviced hospital with skeleton staff was torture. At one point he wished his father would just die but the process took an entire day and the memory still haunts him. Can I ensure that he avoids air hunger?

Back home, his friend got lung cancer and suffered from uncontrollable pain. He still hears his friend's howls in his mind. Does the hospital ever run out of painkillers? What about on the weekend? How does the hospital know that a lot of people suddenly won't need high doses of painkillers? The questions get harder and I fight to prevent my answers from becoming shakier. Does the body adapt to slow starvation, making it harder to die? Does unconsciousness hurt? Could he surface from this deterioration and be forced to live again? What will I write as the cause of his death?

I grip the sides of my chair in amazement. I have never heard a more lucid inquisition into death by a dying man and it is blindingly obvious that he has dwelt on these issues for a long time, turning them over in his mind and perfecting them for a day like today. Entranced, I lose myself in the labyrinth of his words, because as much as they express doubt, I realise that they are also his catharsis. And mine.

Outside, the daily business of the hospital continues. A panicky voice trembles as it declares a cardiac arrest; an intern cajoles a nurse to insert a catheter; a demented man wanders off the ward again.

I feel uncomfortable that I, who cannot help him live, am readily entertaining his death. I keep one eye on the door, as if to avoid getting caught for discussing death when my duty is to save lives. But gradually, as our conversation unfolds, he relaxes and I feel at ease.

As I sit before Mr Vinjic, I reflect how partial doctors are to terms such as 'fix', 'cure' and 'conquer'. The medical student counts a successful rotation as one with procedures. How many intravenous lines or chest tubes did she get to watch? Did anyone let her do any simple tasks? The resident and registrar are triumphant when they clinch a diagnosis; the attending consultant likes nothing more than an efficient ward round of patients whose problems are 'sorted'. Absent from this narrative of professional development is a cohesive way in which to deal with the disappointment, frustration and the plethora of emotions that accompany our perceived failure at conquering disease and suffering.

Had Mr Vinjic needed consent for a procedure, many doctors would have been willing and even the medical student would have been pushed to have a turn, but when it came to talking about his inevitable death, the reluctance was all too real. Part of the reluctance stems from the perceived lack of expertise in having such conversations, hence the 'funny look' from the surgeon and the offer of sending someone who knew how. However, doctors are also poor at accommodating the notion of not being in control.

But what I am most surprised at is the length of time it has taken me to search for an answer to Mr Vinjic's problem, when I knew from the time I read the consult sheet that there wasn't one. I am surprised at how unnerving I find the concept that even in this age, medicine cannot always deliver wonders, yet what I found hardest of all was casting aside my own reluctance to discuss the details of his dying. How ironic that we, witnesses to life in all its glory and ruin, have yet to come full circle and talk easily about death.

I teach my residents that as the population ages, there will be many patients of the likes of Mr Vinjic, who will need our guidance about end of life issues. They will place their trust in us, their oncologist, to discuss matters that may be anathema to others. And the task for us is to learn to do something that does not come naturally to us, for we would rather enthuse about a new therapy than entertain morbid thoughts about death.

I leave his bedside only after ensuring that there is nothing else he wants to know.

'No,' he reassures me with a weak smile, 'there won't be even one more question. This conversation has taken it out of me, but I feel it has been the most meaningful.'

'I will be back tomorrow to check on you anyway,' I say. 'So write down anything you forgot to ask!'

He dies in the middle of the night. The nurse finds him asleep, just the way she settled him into bed after a dose of morphine for pain. He asked her to remove his intravenous line for the night as the beeping interfered with his sleep.

'But you have had it every other night,' she observed.

'And I haven't slept well on a single one. Humour me.'

To her credit, she did.

There was no laboured breathing, no distress calls for pain and no drifting in and out of consciousness, all the things that he had been afraid of. His wife is tearful but accepting of his death, realising that it means an end to watching him suffer with unbearable grace.

I glance at the death certificate the intern has signed. Cause of death – metastatic gastric cancer. These barren words form a poor epitaph to his extraordinary life.

18

◇

My wife does not know

I take a deep breath as I finish the first part of the conversation. 'I will stop now and let you ask me some questions.'

I look at my watch. At twelve p.m. he knew only that the hospital doctors had done a biopsy of his liver and he was here to see me for the results. While at the photocopier, I overhear him speaking to the clerk at the desk.

'Good morning, madam. I am here to see the doctor.'

'We have two different clinics going on. Which one?'

'I don't know, madam,' he answers politely.

'It could be orthopaedics or oncology.' She is too busy jabbing at the computer keyboard to look up.

'Madam, I was only told to come here and I apologise for any confusion. You may wish to wait until my daughter arrives. She probably possesses this information. I gather you expect me to know this.'

The clerk is not used to such reverent patients. I am not used to such immaculate English. She and I look up simultaneously. His daughter has arrived from the parking lot.

'Baba, here is your letter,' she says, handing it over the counter.

'Oncology,' reads the clerk, her expression instantly softening.

'I will take him,' I offer, and escort the man and his daughter into my office.

Now, at twelve forty-five p.m. he knows that he has cancer of the pancreas, that it is advanced and not curable, that he needs chemotherapy for it, and that his chances of long-term survival are poor. He has witnessed and handed out countless weighty decisions in his own career, his words changing the lives of many, but this pronouncement is his alone. How will he reckon with it?

He rubs his chin thoughtfully and asks, 'Doctor, so tell me, when can I return to work? I have a lot to do.'

His eyes light up at the mention of work and he is not focused on my grimace.

'Mr Fareed, I don't think you should travel yet.'

'Why? I feel fine.'

'You may want to have chemotherapy. And even if not, I am not sure what sort of medical backup will be available in Afghanistan if you fall ill.'

'I see.' After a pause, he starts again. 'But there is so much work to do. Everyone in my office is waiting for me to get back.'

At seventy years of age, Mr Fareed has had an illustrious career as a judge and philanthropist in Afghanistan. His list of achievements is long and impressive. He has resettled his family in Australia to escape the war but has maintained an office and a one-room apartment in his home town, several hours travel by bus from the capital. He arrived here one month ago to spend the summer vacation with his wife and four adult children. One night, after experiencing severe chest pain, he was taken to hospital by ambulance with a suspected heart attack. At his age, with his sporadically treated blood pressure, untreated cholesterol and weight creeping up, he had been warned more than once of this possibility and he felt a little sheepish now that the doctor's prediction had come true. But the tests cleared him of a heart attack. Then, as he was about to be discharged, he was gripped by strong pain which led to an urgent CT scan. This detected, completely unexpectedly, an abnormality in his pancreas associated with multiple tumours in the liver. He was admitted to the ward for a liver biopsy, which took three days to arrange. He found the process maddening because no one wanted to tell him exactly what the problem was. It took three days to get a biopsy.

'Probable cancer of the pancreas with liver metastases,' his hospital discharge summary before me blandly states. 'Referred to oncology.'

'Doctor, I must return to work this week. Our elections are coming up.'

'Baba, the doctor just said that you need chemotherapy.'

'Hmm . . . I heard her.' He strokes his chin again.

Mr Fareed looks younger than his seventy years. He is impeccably dressed in a black suit and crimson tie, as if attending a doctor's appointment is no less important than delivering a much-anticipated decision in court. He is clean shaven but has a respectable head of salt and pepper hair that has begun to thin in parts. Somehow, his less than average height emphasises his entire mien as being that of a man with substance and authority.

'So what do you think?' he asks her.

The eldest of his four children, she must be in her early forties. She is wearing a traditional *salwar kameez*, her head respectfully covered with a shawl. She has listened carefully to everything I have said and jotted down notes without interrupting.

'My daughter is a doctor,' Mr Fareed says grandly.

'Oh!' I say, feeling self-conscious.

'I don't work now,' she says in a hasty bid to reassure me. 'I was a doctor in Afghanistan. It seems such a big job to retrain, especially as I am trying to get my kids settled into high school.'

'I understand,' I answer sympathetically. I have met many expatriate female doctors like her who have found the process of starting again just too onerous.

We return to the topic at hand.

'Baba, you should have some chemotherapy.'

He says to me, 'Doctor, I am in your hands and if you feel I need it, I will have treatment. But I ask you to be quick.'

I wince at his apparent naivety. 'Mr Fareed, I can't make the chemo go quicker. It will still be a few months before you can travel and only if you are well enough.'

'Okay, okay! Insha'Allah, God willing.' He joins his hands in submission.

He defies every known toxicity of the treatment he receives.

'What nausea? What tiredness?' he guffaws. 'My job in Afghanistan causes more stress than your therapy!'

He repeatedly asks if he can go back home as he hasn't told his staff about his diagnosis. My answer is always the same.

His mid-treatment scan shows an excellent response to the chemotherapy, with the disappearance of a few tumour spots and shrinkage in others. And in an inspired finish, the post-treatment scan looks dramatically better. Two days later, he wants to get on a flight.

'How long do you intend to be away for?'

'Until next summer.'

You don't have that long, I want to warn. 'Perhaps you could return for a few weeks and tie up loose ends,' I say instead.

'My country needs me.'

Lofty as his aspirations are, he simply doesn't realise that he is unlikely to be able to serve his country in any significant capacity for too much longer.

He plays a frustrating game of cat and mouse with me.

'Well, I am in your hands, doctor.'

'I think you should cut back on travelling.'

'I need to keep working. My country is in the process of rebuilding – it needs all the help it can get.' It is an assertion that several of my Afghan patients make and this time, his perseverance wins over my caution. He spends a happy three months in Afghanistan before I receive a call from his daughter.

'My father is back with a lot of pain. Can we see you?'

'Sure.'

Mr Fareed arrives, not looking as unwell as I had feared.

'I have this nagging pain on my right.'

'We need to get a scan and some blood tests,' I say. 'The pain is coming from your liver.'

'Okay, when?'

'This week.'

'I am going back to Afghanistan tomorrow.'

I grit my teeth in exasperation. 'Mr Fareed, what's the point of doing the scan then?'

'Is it important?'

'Yes!'

I look at his daughter for support. She moves her chair away from her father's line of vision and rolls her eyes at him.

'Tell me, this city where you work. Is there a hospital there? Are there doctors?'

'They do the best they can.'

I spare a thought for the doctors in Afghanistan who may be forced to look after a sick man without having the necessary drugs or equipment to help. Although they will know what needs to be done, in a country hamstrung for resources, their knowledge would be a mere temptress.

His complacency is infuriating. I am close to throwing up my hands but there is something very likeable about the man. He could be anyone's favourite grandfather, a good-natured creature of habit, content to stick to what has worked for him over the years.

I try one last approach, keeping in mind his daughter's presence. 'What does your family think?'

'My daughter has been with me throughout this journey,' he answers, looking at her.

Observing the cultural context, I am sure that his daughter will never dare to publicly cross his wishes. I wish she would. I wish she would tell him as a doctor that his move could be foolhardy; I wish she had a more vocal opinion about some of his less sensible ideas, but if she does, she is not about to share them with me.

'Mr Fareed, what about your wife? What does she want you to do?'

'My wife? She is behind me the whole time.'

'Knowing that you have advanced cancer?'

'Oh, she doesn't know that.'

'She doesn't know that it hasn't disappeared?'

'She doesn't know I have cancer. . .'

I drop my pen with a clatter. 'What do you mean?'

Either he does not notice or chooses to disregard my shriek.

'My wife does not know.'

I look at his daughter for confirmation. She is nodding her head in agreement with her father.

I hold a fistful of his notes in my hand. He has been seeing me for six months!

'What have you told your wife?'

'Not much. She thinks I am having an infection treated.'

'And if you were to die suddenly?'

'Then she would be satisfied that it was destiny and not some disease.'

I look at him incredulously but it is clear from his mild expression that he does not see any incongruity in his statement. For a moment, I am taken aback by the sheer audacity of a husband who would deceive his wife in such a fashion. This is not a matter *like* life and death; it actually *is* life and death.

'Don't you think she might like to know?'

'She is a devout lady. It would worry her too much. I tell her things on a need to know basis.'

Unlike some patients who look for counsel even as they pretend to be convinced about a matter, he appears content with his decision.

His complacency takes my breath away. Cancer patients commonly indicate that one of their greatest needs – often unmet – is for sufficient information which they can then relay to their loved ones. But here is a well-educated, insightful and communicative man, with a daughter who was once a practising doctor – and they are colluding to hide the diagnosis of cancer from their wife and mother respectively. His assertion turns conventional wisdom on its head.

Mr Fareed wins again. He leaves for Afghanistan and proves my worries wrong for another two months. From there, he travels to the United States on official business. It is from there that I receive his next call.

'I don't feel too well, doctor. They say it may be pneumonia,' says a distant voice on the phone.

'Mr Fareed, you can't just keep travelling all over the world expecting to be fine!' I remonstrate with him. I sound like an over-protective mother chiding her child in advance of a misdeed.

He flies back in the next few days and returns to my office, along with his daughter. He has lost some weight and looks haggard, but still not as bad as I had feared. He decides to have the scan he ought to have had some months ago. It reveals the tumour spots in his liver to have grown sizeably along with some new lesions in the lungs. 'Low volume lung disease and unlikely to cause immediate symptoms,' the radiologist's report reckons. But I know that the finding marks another turning point in his journey.

'The cancer has spread, Mr Fareed.'

'Oh.' His right hand travels to his chin.

His daughter's face turns white. 'What do we do now?'

Judging by the burden of his disease and his appearance, further chemotherapy would be futile. 'Tell your wife,' I want to say to him.

'Is there another medicine or chemotherapy I can try?'

Even though many patients realise in retrospect that further chemotherapy did not achieve its promise, it is not always easy to dissuade them from taking this route. My hesitation now is twofold. For Mr Fareed, the problem with accepting that there is no other useful treatment is that he then has to confront his mortality. For me, the problem with letting him accept this conclusion is the diminutive voice in my head that wants to argue that he could be the next Lance Armstrong. All my experience says that he should not enter another round of therapy but how can I be certain of his individual outcome if he does? Are his tumour cells as remarkable as the man they afflict? Will they again melt away with chemotherapy, alarmed by his refusal to let them breed? Or will they follow their usual pattern and make a mockery of the man who would beat his disease into submission?

A training session from my Fulbright year in Chicago floats back to me. The scenario was of a middle-aged man who had progressive cancer but kept insisting on having more treatment. His doctor felt that further treatment was inappropriate and not supported by current evidence. But the man would not listen. The doctor and the patient argued back and forth. The role-players were trained actors, so real that their volleys were discomfiting.

'Is he not listening or is he trying to tell you something?' the lecturer boomed. 'Is the patient misguided or is the doctor plain wrong? Someone tell me what we do now.' We sat with our mouths agape, electrified by the exchange. Finally, the lecturer relented. 'This is a common problem you will encounter every day in your practice and this is how you deal with it.'

The wait for his wisdom seemed interminable.

'You have to find out the hidden agenda! You have to dig for the deeper meaning! Why does Mr Smith want to keep having toxic treatment? Because I tell you, it's not for the sake of having another scan!' Bringing his tone down to a bare whisper, the lecturer continued, 'You, his doctor, have to figure out the reason, because only when you know the reason can you arrive at a solution. Is it his son's graduation or his daughter's wedding that he is desperate to make it to? Is it his golden wedding anniversary or the birth of his first grandchild? Find out what drives your patient. Ask him, "Why do you want to live longer?"'

Although the lecture resembled a frenzied sermon, I eagerly accepted it, and I soon found out that his first assertion was right – the problem did occur on a regular basis. But I also realised that there was no single explanation for a patient's desperate fight to live. Yes, it could be the upcoming graduation, anniversary or birth. Or it could be the holiday or retirement. But there was something else much bigger at play – man's intrinsic hunger to live simply for the sheer joy of being alive. Yes, some of it was unpalatable and downright drudgery, but still, it was the drudgery of life, and it sure beat the anonymity of death.

'There is always something else you can try, but to be honest,

I don't think it will help. And you will still be exposed to the usual side effects.'

I have observed that the most difficult times within oncology consultations do not arise during tense discussions, but in moments of silence. There is rarely anything soothing in the silence that descends like a shroud over the conversations when the news is bad, the diagnosis final, the prognosis devastating. The quiet magnifies my own raucous thoughts and doubts while I sense the same happening to the patient's questions, wishes and fears. And when the silence finally breaks, we each rush to reassure, individually plagued.

Mr Fareed simply stares at the wall. I can see him thinking hard and calculating quickly.

'I am in your hands, doctor.'

I wince at the double-edged sword. What he wants is for me to be the doctor who carries out his will.

'I have mentioned my feelings about more chemotherapy,' I say.

'What else can you do then, if not chemotherapy?'

'Ensure that you are pain-free and comfortable, and call the airline to ban you from flying!'

He smiles feebly at my joke. 'So this is serious.'

It always has been. He just chose not to acknowledge it.

'Yes, I am afraid.'

Large tears begin to fall from his daughter's eyes. Her lip quivers.

'Oh come on, silly girl,' he says to her. 'What's the need to cry?' His voice is damp with the weight of unshed tears.

Suddenly, I feel angry. I realise that while father and daughter sit commiserating, his wife still has no idea of his condition. I feel cheated on her behalf. He has told me that she has been his wife since they were both sixteen years old, wedded in a traditional tribal ceremony, full of pomp and celebration. Their marriage may have been arranged but not the subsequent decades they have spent together, entwined in each other's lives. She has borne him four loving children, tended the household and been the steadfast rock that has allowed him to expand his horizons and come to professional prominence. In turn, he has loved her and provided for her in two countries. How can he not warn her of the adversity that lies ahead?

I know that it is not the most appropriate moment to convince a principled man of his folly, but with my eyes fixed on writing notes, I ask casually, 'Will you tell your wife?'

'Oh, I don't think so. What is the point now?'

I put aside my notes, trying hard to pretend that his decision is immaterial to me. But it is one close to my heart because I have seen it go horribly wrong before. My grandfather never got over the shock of finding out the truth about his wife's cancer. Although he bade her a brave and touching farewell, those who saw him in the months afterwards said he lost his zeal for life and lived each day as a burden. Occasionally, he was heard to lament that he had not had enough time to spend saying his goodbyes. And when, a few months later, he died, his death was a kind of relief for our family, who had seen this once proud man worn out by grief.

Of the many things that elude cancer patients, the most important is certainty. Cancer thrives on doubt, the very mention of it enough to reorder one's way of life. How many vexed patients have I seen, wandering the halls of the hospital from one doctor to another, armed only with the knowledge that someone thinks their trouble may be due to cancer? It is the same with doctors who, once having entertained the diagnosis of cancer, find it unsettling until they can either confirm or banish their suspicion. It seems a cruel irony that on the rare occasion that I know what to do, the patient wants to disregard my opinion. Time is running out and the queue of those who patiently await their turn is growing.

What constitutes a doctor's obligation to a patient, I wonder, and does the covenant sometimes extend beyond the patient to those who are so intimately affected by the patient's condition? As human beings, both doctors and patients have their share of errors, of commission and omission. I know that I am Mr Fareed's doctor, answerable only for the decisions I make regarding his treatment. But I can't beat back my feeling that his case will remain unfinished until his wife knows.

Counselling patients is a fraught business. You try to do what is right for them but so often, you also end up doing what is right for you.

'Mr Fareed, please hear me out. I have met a few patients like you who want to hide their cancer from their spouse. In my experience, the spouse suspects a serious problem and inevitably finds out. This usually happens without preparation, such as if you are visited at home by a nurse or suddenly taken to the emergency room. The patient's initial wish to protect others turns out to be a miscalculation.'

He listens with maddening politeness before getting up from his seat.

'Thank you, doctor. I think I will go for some more treatment.'

I know he considers my warnings mere anecdotes, like the stories people tell about car crashes while using a phone or nudging just over the speed limit. But faced with his intransigence, I have moved to insure my conscience against future regret. I don't feel better but I feel done, for now.

Mr Fareed starts on a second course of chemotherapy. It achieves nothing. Within weeks, he ends up in hospital. The registrar looking after him calls me.

'He has lost a lot of weight and doesn't look good at all. We cannot manage his pain with tablets.'

I advise the registrar to start a syringe driver, a portable drug-delivery device that infuses small but regular amounts of painkillers.

'That sounds like a good idea to keep him comfortable,' he responds with relief. I promise to come and see Mr Fareed the next day.

Early the next morning, I receive a frantic call from the usually cool registrar.

'Mr Fareed's wife is beside herself and won't stop yelling at us. She says we are killing her husband!'

My first question is, 'How is he doing?'

'We finally got him comfortable on the driver.'

Next I ask, 'Why is his wife so upset?'

'When she came in, I sat her down and said that her husband's cancer was terminal. She insisted that no one had ever told her any of this.'

'Did she know that he had cancer?'

'She seemed to know that her husband was having treatment for something, but that's all I could gather.'

'Is her daughter there? She is a doctor.'

'I have seen her and she seems really nice. But she looked anxious, and maybe, a bit burdened. I also don't think she wanted to cross her mother.'

He has interpreted the dynamics accurately.

'So what's happening now?'

His voice quakes. 'Look, I am sorry, it's probably my fault, but I showed her about four letters that you have written, mentioning in all of them your concerns about his advanced cancer and the futility of further therapy. It was then that she lost the plot. We had to call security to restrain her because she attacked the intern. This is my first experience with such things. Does this happen commonly?' I can hear the pleading in his voice.

'No, but it can be traumatic for everyone when it does. You did the right thing.'

Grateful for the support, he tells me that Mr Fareed's wife has been escorted off the hospital premises, while hurling abuse at the staff.

'What do I do now?'

'Concentrate on the patient's best interest.'

This stopgap measure seems like the most appropriate to offer the hapless registrar while I sit at my desk clutching my head in both hands. I knew it, I groan to myself. I knew it. This is one script that follows itself faithfully the few times it happens. It leaves in its wake a trail of bitter recriminations, heartbreaking sorrow and sour memories for all concerned.

A few hours later, I circle the hospital in search of parking. It is close to dusk and as I peer through my windscreen, I think I can make out a familiar figure that I can't quite place before it recedes behind a tree.

Snatching the only available spot, I gather my belongings and walk to the ward. The registrar's agitation is almost palpable.

'Mrs Fareed just walked in, disconnected her husband from the driver, and took him home!'

'But I thought he was sedated.'

'He was but she shook him awake and demanded that he come home with her.'

'Did he say anything?'

'Only to let her do what she wanted.'

I realise that it was Mr Fareed's figure that I briefly spotted downstairs. It is too late now although I doubt I could have changed anything a few minutes ago. I turn to the dismayed registrar who has probably sworn off oncology as a future career.

'Sometimes these things happen despite our best efforts,' I console him.

'We did all we could.'

Although shaken, he seems relieved that he has not committed an unpardonable sin by showing her my correspondence in order to convince her.

I leave, but the problem with Mr Fareed is far from resolved. Together with the charge nurse and other senior staff, we debate over what course of action to take now. Should we call her at home? Should we send the police or the ambulance after him? After much discussion, we elect to let them be, fearing that any more efforts on our part will be perceived as persecutory by his wife.

I think about Mr Fareed all weekend. I think of the genial man who first came to see me, and the fascinating insight into the political landscape of his home country that he would provide from time to time. I looked forward to his visits because he brought images of an unfamiliar land to my doorstep. I think of his remarkable resilience through treatment as well as his respect for his work and staff, even though he had every excuse not to return to work at all. I think of his immaculate presentation to the last and his unwavering politeness. And although I feel upset about his refusal to follow my last request of him, I have always known that it is not personal, because he has expressed his respect and approval of me on several occasions.

Several days pass and then I tempt fate again. Not having found his name in the obituaries, and unable to reach Mr Fareed on his mobile phone, I call his house.

'Are you sure you want to do this?' the secretary asks, raising her eyebrows. News from the ward to the office travels fast.

'Yes, he is still my patient,' I answer, not willing to share my trepidation.

As if to continue the debacle with a vengeance, Mrs Fareed answers the phone. I don't introduce myself but ask if I can speak to her husband.

'Who are you?' she asks, her tone steeped in suspicion.

'The oncologist looking after your husband.' I want to emphasise the present tense.

'What do you want?'

'I am calling to see if he is okay.'

The floodgates open. She lets out a primitive howl of rage that flies down the phone before revealing the most spectacular repertoire of abuse that I have ever witnessed. I am breathless, always having cast her in my mind as a simple village woman with little or no command of English. Without paying any attention to the silence on the other end of the line, she curses me for labelling her husband with a disease he did not have, for giving orders to kill him with morphine and for colluding with the doctors and nurses to withhold information from her. He is alive, she crows triumphantly. He is alive, despite what I tried to do to him. Filling her lungs with air, the final words she roars probably encapsulate her salient observation about the medical profession in general, and me in particular: 'You are all evil. One day, you too will get what is owed to you!'

There is no point in trying to break through the fog of invective. Although I am glad that he is alive, I long to know how he is doing. I want to know that he is comfortable because pain has been a prominent part of his suffering and it does not have to be so. But there is a part of me that simply wants to know that *he* knows it is not how she says it is. I imagine him caught in an awkward situation, having to either defend his untruths or profess his ignorance. I groan at the unpleasantness of either.

After seeing him so much over six months, I also feel entitled to an opportunity to say a better goodbye. But part of being a doctor is dealing with the unfairness of the demands placed upon us in the heat of the battle and reminding ourselves that the battle is against the disease and not the doctor. It is about cataloguing encounters so that when incidents such as this jar, there are others to cushion the fall. It is time to move on from perceived wrongs. I have been the proxy for the disease that Mr Fareed's family could not see or touch. I may have shed some pride but her loss is everlasting.

19

◇

Please stay

It is a glacial Sunday morning in winter. Judging by the silence in the trees and on the roads, even the birds have agreed to sleep in a little longer. The cloudless sky has made for a bitterly cold night; there is a powder of frost on the grass and on the windscreen of our cars, which had to be left outside the garage because I misplaced the remote door-opener yesterday. I recoil from the bright kitchen light and simultaneously groan at the fluorescent green time on the microwave. It is five twenty-nine a.m. This is the sixth consecutive morning either my husband or I have had to roll groggily out of bed to attend to the hunger pangs of our one and a half year old daughter, who, her doctor says, is making up for lost time because severe reflux prevented her from eating properly for the first twelve months. I think grumpily that once fed, she will return satisfied to her warm cot, while it will be too late for me to recapture a peaceful sleep. This leads to the even more disagreeable thought that there is not even a hypothetical option to make up for lost sleep today, as I am due at work. In turn, I am reminded that this is my third consecutive weekend of working. At five twenty-nine a.m., everything seems unfair.

At six-thirty a.m. it feels like our entire household has been awake for hours. My daughter defies my prediction and omits her second sleep; my three-year-old son wants to know why, waking up my sleep-deprived husband in the process. Downstairs, the peals of laughter that ring out from among a mountain of toys do little to energise either of us as, between yawns, we contemplate the long day ahead. There is a swimming lesson to attend, a birthday party and then a family dinner to host. At six-thirty a.m., everything seems disagreeable.

And as if the heavens had divined this morning to be one fit for argument, we discover that we have run out of milk! The thought of enduring the winter chill on an already violated Sunday morning is enough to lead to the exchange of frosty, accusatory glances from behind the newspaper as we wait for each other to do the honourable thing and offer to get the milk. As he walks out with deliberate steps, I wish that I had gone instead because numerous pieces of Lego have just crashed in a heap at my feet. My daughter, a novice to walking, slips, lands amidst them and lets out a mighty howl at the indignity of it all.

'This is so ordinary,' my husband mutters. At seven-thirty a.m. as I wave goodbye to the family, it suddenly doesn't sound like such a bad idea to be going to work! Defrosting the windshield is the hardest part of getting there, as the roads are well clear of anyone who does not have to be outdoors.

This is my weekend at the hospice. The charge nurse greets me enthusiastically; we have known each other for years and I like her not only for her kind manner but also her ability to distinguish the neediest people in a house full of seriously ill patients. As I rummage through my bag for a pen, she volunteers, 'They are mostly pretty quiet today. You should be able to get home quickly.' She has three young children and is sympathetic to my weekend commitments.

Such can be the power of suggestion that just hearing these words makes me feel better about my prospects.

'Okay, run me through the list,' I say.

We go down the freshly printed list by bed numbers. The man in bed one has picked up and may fulfil his wish of getting home. The lady in bed two needs a transfusion and the one in bed four is comfortable. Beds seven and nine need their painkillers adjusted and bed sixteen wants a sleeping pill and laxatives. A handful of patients are unconscious and expected to die within the next day.

'Bed twenty is dying. I don't think you need to see her.'

'What's wrong with her?' I ask, scanning my list. Nina Rogers is listed as thirty years old. I vaguely recall the handover from a weary colleague at the end of what had been a tense week of work for her. But running through the long list of patients, her details had merged with those of the others and if there had been a word of warning or emotion in her voice, it was not immediately obvious to me.

The nurse shakes her head. 'She has breast cancer and got sick two weeks ago.'

'What happened?' I ask curiously.

She shrugs. 'I am not sure, but anyway, there is nothing to do now.' I tell myself that her measured tone is probably a simple acceptance of what she has seen unfolding every day and I move on to the first patient.

True to the nurse's assertion, the patients prove to be an easy lot. Of those who are awake, some are picking at their breakfast and assure me that they are being well taken care of. There are the usual requests for laxatives, a glass of beer and a sign outside the door to limit visitors. 'It is easier if the doctor says so,' a woman explains between hard-earnt breaths. A Mandarin-speaking gentleman holds up a sign that says 'Doctor, call daughter.' I tap at my watch, indicating it's too early, but he just shakes his head vigorously. I call her to answer her questions, all simple. In between seeing patients, I rewrite drug charts and fill out fluid orders, ticking off each task as I go. I keep waiting to strike a difficult patient, a vexed family member or a knotty problem. But the patients seem content, it is too early for visitors, and if there were any problems, the previous doctor had solved them.

I linger outside the last room, bed twenty, where Nina Rogers is dying – comfortably, I am assured. Should I check on her or let her be? I look at my watch. It is just before eleven a.m. and if I left now, I could take my son to the much-anticipated birthday party. But the very thought of leaving a patient unseen to make it to a social occasion seems untoward. On the other hand, the nurse has specifically stated that this patient does not need to be seen by a doctor and there is no reason to disregard her. I stand quietly at the door for a full minute, debating the difference between being intrusive and thorough. A word either way would convince me. I curse the gullibility of my conscience, which seeks to enter into arguments with itself at inopportune moments.

I knock lightly, almost inaudibly, at the door, deciding that to break habit is unnecessary. Not expecting to receive an invitation, I open one half of the double doors and tiptoe in. Checking on Nina will take a few seconds, I tell myself, having briefly flicked through the sad essentials of her notes, and I can then be on my way home with an easy conscience.

I nearly jump out of my skin as I look up, for there, surrounding Nina's bed, are at least half a dozen people. I feel like an animal caught in the glare of a car's headlight. From a cursory look at them, I can see that things are going badly and I try to extract myself from the situation with some propriety.

'Good morning. I am the doctor on today. I wanted to make sure Nina was okay.' The nurse had already told me she was, but for some reason I needed to see for myself.

No one speaks. The answer is obvious, they seem to say. It depends on what you mean by okay.

Wishing to avoid awkwardness by turning back now, I deliberately move toward Nina's bed. In the few steps it takes to get there, my first impression is that of a little girl peacefully asleep in bed. Underneath the sheets, her frame is svelte and long. Her skin is like porcelain; her face, a stranger to wrinkles. Dark brown lashes rest against high-rising cheekbones. Her lustrous hair is brushed back from her face, neatly fanned on the pillow.

I stand at the end of her bed and watch her breath rise and fall. She looks as if she could wake up any moment, yawn lazily and exclaim, 'Oh my God! What time is it?!' Then I turn to the relatives in the room, four of whom have discreetly slipped out.

'How is she doing?' I ask the lady who is obviously Nina's mother.

'Okay,' she shrugs lightly. Then more inquisitively, 'What do you think?'

'She looks peaceful.' I am lost for another neutral description.

I look at the patient some more.

'How are you doing?' I ask the man on the other side. He is young, like her. Dark shadows line his unshaven face. He has not left her side for days. It must be hard to watch his sister dying, I think. He looks away.

My choices appear again. Satisfied she is comfortable, I could leave. But I can both sense and smell the air of sadness that pervades the room and where there is such sadness there is usually the need to talk: I should stay and see.

In response to my wandering eye, her mother says, 'We are religious people as you can tell.'

'Religion can be an important anchor in such times,' I agree, nodding at the prayer books and icons that line the mantelpiece.

'There is nothing else left but to believe in a miracle.'

I silently and sadly acknowledge that she is right. I know from her notes that only five years ago, Nina discovered a lump in her breast after she returned from an extended holiday in Europe. Despite the temptation to ignore it, she decided to check with her doctor, who diagnosed her with breast cancer. The next week, Nina was having a mastectomy followed by the recommended chemo-therapy and radiotherapy. Then, she developed a secondary cancer in the brain. Her respite after neurosurgery was brief before more lesions became evident. For the past three years, she has undergone several operations and other gruelling therapy. But finally, when the last tumour appeared, her doctors threw up their hands. Despite this, Nina kept up her hopes and submitted herself to complemen-tary medicine in the form of injections and special diets, perhaps herself believing they would help, but also to console her family. But her health continued to fail. The final insult came one week ago when she suddenly collapsed. Her family agreed it was time for hospice care.

As I look at Nina's mother, I see a woman in the prime of her life, a mother who had her children young. She caresses her daughter's hand, telling me that she has not left the room since they arrived.

'I promised my daughter that I would stay with her,' she says, tears streaming down her tired face. 'I just wish she could talk. I just wish she could hear me.'

In that instant, unbidden images of my own children flash before my eyes and I experience a pain as if my own heart is breaking. For me, the forlorn figure of a mother presiding over a dying child is the most gut-wrenching, confronting and sobering aspect of being a doctor. Each time I witness it, I am despondent for days, questioning the fairness of life, the existence of a higher power that somehow considers this just, and the point of being a doctor converted to a helpless bystander.

'Does your daughter have children?' I ask, silently hoping the answer is no.

'No.'

'That's a relief,' are the first words that spring from my lips. The most painful separations that I have witnessed, the ones that unsettle me to the core, are those involving mother and child. I no longer need to imagine in order to empathise, with children of my own.

'Yes and no,' answers the young man. 'We were trying to have a baby when she got diagnosed.'

I kick myself for assuming she was single.

'I am sorry. I didn't mean to be insensitive. I can leave now.'

'Please stay,' they both request simultaneously. The quiet wait for death must be unbearable.

I feel light-headed as I pull up a chair. An intense wave of nausea rises from the depth of my body and I feel chilly, sweaty and nervous all at once. It is like being thoroughly unprepared for a crucial exam on which your life depends. I don't want to be in the room, for though I am closer to the patient in age, I feel at one with the mother. And surrounded by so much sadness, it is only a matter of time before my mind will start playing its gory tricks on me. In such situations, I have often wistfully wondered what it would be like to possess a more resilient skin that would simply deflect the sadness back to its owner, instead of absorbing it and allowing it to seep through my being, bruising a feeling here, pinching a nerve there. But what sort of a doctor would I be then, present in body yet absent in soul? And what kind of care would I provide to my patients? A generic, one size fits all kind of care that is as sterile as the words in my chemotherapy protocol book?

What would keep me awake at night if not the dilemmas of life and death and what would I tabulate my blessings against? When I think of these possibilities, I want to hold on to every bit of my 'feeling' self, despite the occasional challenges. For I know that this, to me, is the essence of being a doctor.

I know she would understand if I said I was busy or that I find it too sad to be in the room. But it takes a mere pause to remember that it is an extraordinary privilege to be allowed into the final phase of a stranger's life. And being a doctor demands sacrifices that sometimes reach beyond working late hours and missing a meal or two.

'I will stay here as long as you need me to.' I am surprised and a little disappointed at how deeply I have to draw on my emotional reserve to make this straightforward offer.

A thick blanket of cloud casts a dark shadow across what should have been a light-filled afternoon. The mother lights a candle to illuminate the room and chants a prayer. We all bow. Nina has not moved once, perhaps listening in on the supplication.

Her mother sprinkles some water over her pillow. 'My friend brought in this holy water. She said it's famous for curing cancer.'

Nina's husband looks on dubiously but politely. It is hard to watch when holy water supersedes modern medicine in the minds of relatives.

Then, without invitation or warning, Nina's mother and husband start to recall her life. I learn about her work as a music teacher, her love of children and her affection for her four older siblings. I learn about her wicked wit and share a laugh at her favourite joke. I hear about the mature and dignified way in which she handled the persistently disappointing pronouncements about her prognosis even as her peers looked happily into their future, the prospect of death not even registering on their young minds.

Nina married young and was very proud of her own house, which she had decorated over the years, but when she fell seriously ill, she asked to return to her childhood home. With her husband, she moved back into the small bedroom that used to be hers, telling him that it made her feel secure in a life that was increasingly filled with uncertainty.

'Like a lot of mothers, I never stopped secretly hoping that my little girl would never leave home. When she came back, I felt sad but so grateful for her kindness to me.' Every morning for the past six months, the entire family joined in for breakfast, Nina's favourite time. It was yet another way, her mother says, of Nina knitting the family together, even as she prepared to leave the fold.

'Every day when I saw her sick I felt as if someone was smashing me into pieces, but I am so glad she allowed us to share her. She could have stayed with her husband but she thought of everybody.'

As I listen, the seemingly minor details of her short life assume real proportions and the woman lying before me goes from being a patient to a person. My reluctance to sit with her changes to an interest in her journey. And, contrary to my fears, my experience of spending time with her grieving family is not distressing as much as revealing.

While Nina's mother recounts the satisfaction of nurturing her child, her husband wants to talk about the last few weeks leading up to hospice. 'What I hated most was seeing her disabled. By the end, you could sense there were pieces of her missing. She forgot her sister's birthday and was angry with herself for days. She would try to talk about her favourite restaurant and could not find the words. "Why is my brain tricking me?" she would scream. "I just want to think straight!"'

She became resigned to her dependence on him to go to the bathroom or walk down the stairs. 'I tried to make a joke of it and say it was just like carrying her over the threshold to our new house all over again,' he smiles.

She asked her oncologist to refer her to a psychiatrist. Her husband enjoys reminiscing about a particular visit to the doctor: 'The oncologist was amazed. He said people twice her age had trouble asking for help and here she was, saying, "I know it is going to happen. Help me prepare."' Nina had even offered to give a talk to medical students about the experience of being terminally ill at a young age.

He looks at Nina again and returns to the present. 'When she collapsed this time and we took her to hospital, they started doing all the tests again, but I told them there was nothing they could do. Two different doctors came back and said, "We have bad news. She is dying." I was desperate to buy Nina some peace so I replied, "I could have told you that if you had listened to me." Sometimes, doctors have a way of behaving as if they are the only ones who know what's right or best for a person. I just wish they would listen to us – I am not a specialist but I know Nina better than any doctor. I wish we hadn't spent a whole day in emergency.'

A day is a long time in the life of a person who only has a few left. 'I am sorry,' I say. 'That sounds stressful and perhaps unnecessary.'

'It's the sort of stuff our minds go back to, probably because we are so helpless,' he reflects. His voice sounds disillusioned and defeatist, yet I can't deny that his words carry a fundamental truth.

Sometimes, in the hustle and bustle of daily medical work, it is easy to forget the person behind the illness. All too often, an unending list of tasks distracts us from meaningful engagement with the patient at the end of life. In this age of modern technology, what patients and their relatives increasingly want from doctors is a return of the old touch, the touch of healing and humanity that seemed to exist in abundance when there was nothing else the doctor could do.

Nina passes away quietly in the early hours of the morning with her family close by. When I return to work, they are still there, maintaining vigil until the funeral director arrives. This time, I find it easier to enter her room although my heart is still heavy. But I want to pay tribute to her family, and her mother in particular, for the remarkable and heart-wrenching journey on which she has accompanied her daughter. Nina lies as peacefully as ever, the only noticeable difference the absent rise and fall of her chest. I have no right words with which to console her mother on this most unthinkable of losses, but I tell her that we should all be grateful that Nina is finally free of pain, suffering and more dashed hopes.

As I leave the room for the final time, her mother follows me out and says quietly, 'Thank you for being there yesterday.' Returning her embrace, I remind myself that sometimes, it is enough to simply stay and listen.

20

◇

Keep peace with your soul

On a morning's rounds, I walk into an intern engrossed at the computer.

'I am looking up all the diseases that Mr Crosby died of.'

The octogenarian had been on our unit for four weeks with multi-organ failure. His usually jovial nature changed in the last few days and we all accepted that he had given up on life. I thought we had a good rapport with his family too so I am somewhat surprised by the wariness implied in the intern's tone.

'Is there a problem?'

'Not yet,' she says. 'But you know what families are like. They will want to know a hundred answers.'

I watch the printer splutter to life and think better of arguing the point. But her warning echoes in my ears all day long.

That evening in the hospital chapel, I anxiously scan the gathering crowd, perhaps also expecting a hundred answers. The minimal conversation is hushed and respectful. I feel my dread creep up with every filling seat. I try to laugh off my indulgent assumption that the room's collective sentiment will soon be directed at me. Yet the air feels thick with grief and sobriety and I feel ambushed.

Two months ago, I accepted a friendly request to speak at the memorial service of our oncology unit. Twice a year, the chaplaincy invites bereaved relatives of cancer patients to join in an ecumenical service. A lot of preparation goes into ensuring that the occasion is appropriate: sensitive yet understated. Having always held the chaplains in high regard, I agreed immediately to help.

Everywhere I look, there are vaguely familiar faces. It is like walking down the street and glimpsing someone whose name is on the tip of your tongue. This room is populated with a hundred such glimpses. I avoid them by looking down at the sheet of names in my hand. Mrs Ali, whose breast cancer finally caught up with her; Mrs James with the undiscovered primary; Luke, who found the melanoma during a cycling tour. There is also Mr Harding, the affable man whom I have known since my resident days. But for every name that tallies with a diagnosis, many more trigger no specific memory. I know something terrible went wrong with Mr Peters. Or was that someone else? Is that his daughter or his second wife? Is that the son who lodged a formal complaint months after his mother died? My snippets of information carry no substance, whereas I once knew everything about these patients. Yet though my recollection has waned, that of the relatives is about to come alive. This audience tonight represents 'the worst of'. It represents suffering, death and loss and the formidable crowd of gathered relatives will view it as our collective failure to save a loved one.

I am at the lectern. As if on cue, the sound of quiet sobbing punctuates the chaplain's introduction. I can't locate her but her sobs will form the backdrop to the entire service. Two children still in school uniform sit quietly at their mother's feet. Young professionals share the rows with the elderly and retired, all in anticipation of what will unfold.

In my sweaty hands, I hold the crumpled remains of the speech I jotted down earlier today. I have realised, too late, that its stiffness and formality is simply wrong for the occasion. But so-called speeches from the heart require emotional investment and as I stand here, I wish I had left myself more time to judge the correct pitch.

I plunge in. 'Thank you for being here tonight. I am not sure that I could have done it if I were in your shoes.' I immediately feel better for having said this. The oncology ward is a stone's throw away – just walking down the corridor would take courage. A daughter in the front row squeezes her mother's hand.

'I want to thank the people who we are here to remember.' Many heads are bowed. I pay tribute to the dignity and fortitude of patients through their illnesses before acknowledging their support network, something that we doctors silently but gratefully count on. A few heads nod appreciatively. Encouraged, I talk about the goodwill of those who undergo gruelling therapy, who wait in our waiting rooms, procedure rooms and many other rooms, none of which provide the comfort of home. In the daily grind of our work, we become enslaved to many simultaneous tasks but deep down, we care about our patients and worry about them. A couple shares a glance; I suddenly remember the brother and sister who took turns to attend appointments with their parents, who were dying simultaneously of lung cancer. They always fretted that we would confuse the details.

I want to stop but I am afraid that if I do, the audience will fill the void with its own questions. Out of the corner of my eye, I see the husband of a young woman who sought desperately for any experimental therapy to buy her time with her children. Pregnant at that time, I had felt particularly strained and disillusioned caring for her. Seeing his woebegone expression compels me to add that medical science is on the march every day to find newer, better treatments for cancer. My eyes well with tears. I stop.

There is a yawning silence in the room. Everyone looks straight ahead. Yet it does not feel awkward. It is as if we all need a moment to collect our thoughts. I am surprised by how moved I am, despite dealing with death and dying on most days. Perhaps this feels different because the urgency of death has faded, leaving in its wake a distillation of all the other emotions that swirl in our mind.

I walk back to my seat and watch as each name is read out and a candle lit in memory of the deceased. Hands tremble as relatives come forward. A wheelchair-bound man progresses thoughtfully up the aisle. The room collectively stops breathing as the two young children respond to their father's name. No one even tries to hide the tears. Then the last name has been read, the last candle lit. The chaplain whispers that I can leave if I like.

Hanging back behind the crowd, I set myself a deliberate challenge. I walk up to the table of photographs, where I see a multitude of faces, all in various poses of vitality – gardening, completing a marathon, playing with a child – before they became cancer patients. I am able to recognise a handful at best. I feel a stab of guilt. I light a candle and reflect on these lost lives. It is hard to imagine them as anything but patients, yet clearly these photographs tell a different story. Battle-hardened as I sometimes feel from the procession of deaths I witness, tonight's service makes me feel sad and reflective.

Outside, I brace myself for the questions that will come as my eyes skim the crowd. I practise the answers. 'Sometimes even young people can get overwhelming infections.' 'I don't think that another cycle of chemotherapy would have helped your daughter.' 'I am sorry that drug had not been approved at the time your husband died.' 'I too wish we had a cure for cancer.'

The wheelchair stops next to me. The old man seems to be speaking into the air when he says, 'It is the weekends that are the worst. I guess that's when we spent time together.' Someone brings him a cup of tea and just as I am about to respond, I see the schoolchildren leaving. I run to catch up with them.

'I just wanted to thank you for coming,' I say, particularly touched by the children's composure.

Their mother looks towards the ward and chokes. Her own mother puts a hand on hers. 'We needed to do this,' she says.

'I am very sorry for your loss,' I offer, furiously trying to recall whether I ever met her husband.

'He died within four weeks of his diagnosis,' the children's mother responds. Is there closure in her words or an implicit accusation?

'We *have* to go,' her daughter says urgently. As she herds her family out, every nuance screams untapped grief, unfinished business.

Next, an elderly woman beams as she recalls a letter that my colleague wrote her on the death of her husband. 'It was the most graceful and elegant letter I have ever read so I put it away with my jewellery in the bank.' I wish he was there to collect the accolade.

A man taps me on the shoulder. 'How are your children, doctor?' I remember in a flash his wife's ritual question to me. Two women hesitatingly tell me that their husbands turned back from the hospital entrance. I reassure them that this is not unusual. People are milling everywhere, absorbing stories and consoling one another, no one wanting to leave.

The next time I look at my watch, two hours have passed and not a single question has been asked of me, not a single reservation expressed about patient care, although I know far too well that there must be many. I feel foolish now but also touched by the generosity that relatives are willing to show those who they associate most closely with their loved one's death. It is a deeply humanising experience and one that I wish the intern from this morning was present to witness. She would have seen that bereaved relatives are not always looking for someone to blame or question.

The practice of medicine turns us into dispassionate observers of death. On a really busy day in clinic, a death or two is greeted with silent relief. An impending death puts into motion plans for the next patient to come in. Hospital administrators refer to deaths as 'negative outcomes' and newspapers flog death statistics to needle governments about their inaction. Anatomy lessons on cadavers are being replaced with virtual images, and the autopsy room is tucked away discreetly at the back of the hospital. Without saying it or perhaps even meaning it, we all get the idea that a patient's death equates to the doctor's failure. We don't pause to reflect on death; indeed, the less we say, the better we are thought to cope.

It would be a glib conclusion that attending a memorial service necessarily makes one a better doctor, as that requires years of painstaking learning, trial and error. I am also not sure that it suddenly transforms one into a more sensitive being because all of us who look after the sick are aware of the enormous responsibility we bear towards our patients. But what the service achieved for me is that in its aftermath, I felt humbled. As I watched a hundred thin candles glow and flicker, guarded by the photographs of people before they became patients, I felt in the presence of a silent but powerful lesson – that we, as doctors, are neither omniscient nor invincible, that the circle of life is all-encompassing. I am sure that our patients would sometimes love to tell us this when we don't listen to them as closely as we should and instead construct our own priorities about what matters to them.

I suspect that in our private moments, we do reflect on the extraordinary privilege and power that accompanies being a physician. But I, like many others, am guilty of forgetting this from time to time. And if it takes a simple and poignant memorial service to make me a more aware physician, then it has probably achieved more than many other compulsory meetings that populate the year's calendar.

It is late at night as I leave. A car is stuck at the boom gates, the driver having run out of change. I let her through using my card. She catches up with me at the traffic lights and, rolling down her window says, 'I wasn't sure about tonight but I am glad I came.' The lights change before I can respond in kind.

As if by some design, the next day I receive a phone call from Tom Cleary's wife, Ivana. It has been just over a month since Tom died of progressive lung cancer and the last time I spoke to Ivana was immediately following his death. I ask her how she is holding up now after the last few testing months.

'I am glad he is at peace,' she offers, 'but it's horribly lonely without him. I think what I miss most is his attitude – he was just so selfless.'

I agree with her wholeheartedly and tell her that I miss seeing Tom too. Not sure of her precise reason for calling me, I ask her if there is anything else I can do for her.

She hesitates before saying, 'Look, you are probably too busy, but I wanted you to know that we are holding a memorial service for Tom this afternoon. I would be delighted if you came. Tom wanted the service as a celebration of his life and I think he would have liked to have you there.'

The invitation catches me completely by surprise and I am touched to be remembered in this way. By the time a patient dies, the journey for everybody concerned has been so arduous that it is understandable when patients wish nothing more to do with the hospital or the oncologist. I have subsequently run into several relatives who have expressed their gratitude and told me that they had always meant to call or write but the task seemed too onerous with the memory still fresh.

'I wanted to personally ask you so I didn't put an invitation in the mail. I will give you the address just in case.'

Tom's face flashes before me. My mind travels from his suave appearance when he first saw me, thinking he had a curable disease, to his unprecedented anguish on his very last visit, when he had felt abandoned. Despite the passage of some time, the latter recollection still makes me uneasy, causing my response to tumble out: 'Ivana, that's very nice of you. I have a tight schedule today and I just don't think I can make it.'

'Oh, that's a shame,' she says, clearly disappointed. 'I should have asked you earlier.'

'I am sorry but it's not your fault. You have enough on your plate.'

'Anyway, thank you for looking after Tom. It's a pity you won't be there to hear what he was really like, because this service is a real celebration, not a mourning.'

I hang up and spend the rest of the morning flustered by this simple conversation. It is true that my day is busy but this is not the real reason for declining the invitation to Tom's service. As his oncologist and as the embodiment of the profession that could not help him, I don't see it as my place to attend such a personal event. Why did Ivana invite me? Was it merely out of obligation or was it Tom's idea? Tom had once indicated that he was making a guest list for the service. Would attending it be a final mark of respect towards him? I feel oddly conflicted and frustrated at my uncharacteristic inability to adhere to a decision.

Sticking to my intended schedule, I leave one hospital bound for another, where a mound of paperwork awaits me. I have been hoarding it for days, waiting for an occasion to dispense with the job. But as I drive, I can't take my mind off Tom's service, due to start in an hour. What will it be like? What sort of people did a man like Tom befriend? Was it really possible to celebrate a life in its passing? At the freeway, I deliberately slow down to allow myself a final chance to decide. Then I switch lanes and drive in the opposite direction to the venue of the service. My determination lasts another few minutes before I exit and pull over in a quiet street. Feeling quite ridiculous by now, I call my husband.

'What would you do?' I ask.

'I would go,' he answers without hesitation. 'Families of dead patients don't really ask much of us.'

'It looks so silly to change my mind.'

'It's not about you.'

His words compel me to turn around, speed home, change into a black dress, and re-enter the freeway with new-found resolve.

The church where Tom and Ivana married is nestled in a beautiful part of the city. It is a resplendent autumn afternoon, the sun shining down from a cloudless, piercing blue sky. Majestic green trees form a wide canopy over the gently winding street. I realise in the instant that I enter the street that the gathering will be large. There is no parking to be found. As I drive past the church, I turn my head to glance at the crowd. A queue of men, women and children is inching towards the front door. I duck into a side street, squeeze my car into the last available spot, and make a dash towards the church. The last thing I want is to draw attention by being late.

From the back of the queue where I smooth down my dress, one of the first things I notice is the riot of colours and the mood that accompanies it. Hardly anyone is wearing black and, however subdued, there is definitely cheer. At the door, Ivana cuts a beautiful figure in a pink suit. The young woman standing beside her could only be Tom's daughter; the resemblance is striking.

A condolence book lies on a table next to the entrance. By the time I reach it, most pages are filled. I notice with relief that there is room only to write my name. I choose to sign with only an illegible signature, smiling as I think that Tom would claim the practice to be customary for doctors.

When I finally reach Ivana, her face breaks into a wide and welcoming smile. 'You made it!' She hugs me and I move on quickly to allow her to greet those behind me. Her daughter is speaking to somebody so I wait. She is lanky like Tom and her facial expressions remind me of her father.

She looks up at me without recognition and I quickly say, 'You must be Tom's daughter.' I kick myself for having forgotten her name. 'My name is Ranjana.'

Still, no recognition. The lady behind me is at my heels. 'I was his oncologist,' I whisper.

'Oh, of course!' she says, gripping my hand. 'Daddy talked about you all the time!'

The lady behind me looks on curiously and I quickly make my way inside.

To hear Tom referred to as Daddy jolts me into remembering the reason for this almost festive gathering. A young girl has lost her father, a woman her husband.

Inside, I find myself a seat in the back row, adjacent to and obscured by an ornate cream-coloured pillar. I am satisfied that it is a place sufficiently discreet. From here, I can watch the people who file in without being observed. A handful of people from both sides of the family usher guests into the pews. Clearly, the people gathered here are mutually familiar; I watch them exchange fond greetings and embraces. So far the back row has been scantily occupied but as people continue to pour in, the seats on either side of me are quickly taken. I avoid making conversation with either stranger by staring straight ahead.

The small dais is filled by a framed photograph of Tom on the day he was married; he was a dashing young man. The camera lens caught him in a pensive moment. He looks reflectively into the distance, poised on the threshold of a new life. Although the Tom I saw was thirty years older and encumbered by disease, the reflective expression did not change. Scattered around the frame are several smaller photographs and a poem whose words I cannot read from my seat. Flowers of all varieties and colours adorn the room. The priest who married the couple opens the service with a short prayer before handing over to Tom's brother, who conducts the rest of the ceremony tearfully but masterfully.

One after another, they step up to the dais. Tom's siblings, who remember their youngest brother as the fairest and the most disciplined of them all. Tom's ageing mother, who, despite her dementia, recognises that in burying her son, she has somehow outlived her welcome on this earth. His many nieces and nephews, who line up together to record their fondest memory of their uncle. 'The time when I was struggling with my job and he said it was okay to follow my dream,' says one. 'The summer I turned seven when he took my pet rabbit to the vet,' say another. And so on, his family recalls the many things that Tom did and the advice he offered, always without pretence, never expecting anything in return. These are the things that stuck in their mind and forever earnt their loyalty.

It is now the turn of Tom's friends. The audience learns that he befriended a group of boys in high school. They went on to finish university together, witness each other's weddings, children, grandchildren and all the momentous occasions in between. They were the men Tom had dinner with the night he died. Some of the men sob openly at having lost the link that united them. The woman to my right starts to cry.

'That's my husband up there. God, this is hard.'

I nod sympathetically.

'How do you know Tom?' she asks, sniffing into her handker-chief. This is the question that I have been dreading.

'I used to be his doctor.'

'Oh, are you Joanna? He has known you for years, right?' she presses.

'I was his oncologist.'

'Oh, oh . . .'

A deep frost descends between us. Her body recoils from me as if my very line of work is contaminating. I tell myself that this is a normal reaction to her feeling cheated of a lifelong friend and I try not to let it bother me. But I can't help noticing that she does not then speak to me for the entire duration of the service.

Tom's daughter speaks. She reads a thoughtful poem she has penned about her memories of her father and her hopes of con-tinuing to make him proud. She reads with the dignity and grace that was Tom's hallmark when he was struggling with cancer. I can understand why he was always bursting with pride when he mentioned his only child. He had harboured apprehensions about his capacity to be a good father – obviously, his fears had been unfounded. As I watch her promise her father that she will care for her mother, I feel sad for her loss in particular. She is far too young to relinquish the leading influence in her life. There is spontaneous applause when she finishes. She stands bravely to acknowledge it. I can't help wondering how much this day will exhaust her.

Ivana has chosen not to speak for fear of not being able to con-tain her sorrow. Instead, her niece reads out a prepared speech in which she recalls the love and inspiration Tom provided in the four decades of their partnership. There is a very personal section about her devastation when he was diagnosed with cancer, balanced by his courage in dealing with the terrible consequences of the disease.

She talks about the good humour with which he underwent the toxic treatments, the maturity with which he accepted their failure and the equanimity with which he met his end. In between the diagnosis and its conclusion, she says, he continued to walk the dog, paint the fence and serve his customers. I realise that although I can attest to the medical details she mentions, I never fully appreciated what a full parallel life he strived for even as the sun set on it.

Ivana thanks a host of people who helped Tom and singles out his family doctor for mention. 'Tom always said that she made him feel safe, as often with her soothing words as her treatments.' I wonder if the doctor is here today to hear this heart-warming description.

When Ivana's statement finishes to the sound of more applause, classical music starts to play softly in the background. 'It's his favourite compilation,' a woman in front of me whispers to her neighbour.

I look around me to see whether this is the end of the ceremony, when Tom's best friend returns to the dais. As if in a rush to start, he says, 'Ladies and gentlemen, this is going to be particularly hard. Before Tom died, he wrote a letter and he asked me if I would read it at his memorial service. I immediately said yes and ever since then, I have wondered if I would do him justice. He told me to open it at the service so I beg you to bear with me as I go through with Tom's final request.'

The quiet murmur in the room is replaced with stunned, silent anticipation. I catch the back of Ivana's head, shaking slowly.

He carefully opens the envelope and takes out some sheets of yellow writing paper. He arranges them in order and braces himself to start. Then, he stares closely at the letter and lets out a grin followed by a laugh.

'My dearest family and friends,' he utters gravely. 'The view is fantastic, the food lousy and not a virgin in sight! No email to check, not a phone to be found, no bills to pay. Rest easy, for I am finally at peace.' The words puncture the solemnity of the occasion, reminding me of Tom's other jokes in clinic.

As his friend continues, it is as if Tom is speaking to the congregation. He reveals that the letter has taken him eighteen months and five versions to perfect. I calculate that he must have started writing it at the time of his initial diagnosis. With his trademark grace and maturity, he carries the audience along with what it has been like to live with a death sentence.

'As I have become more disabled, I have become increasingly grateful for your calls and visits that have brought the outside world to my doorstep again. It is this cutting off from the world that I feared the most.'

He thanks his siblings and his wife's family, with whom he clearly shared a strong bond. He expresses regret that this year's family retreat was to be his last but says that he is heartened by the fact that these retreats provided him with more happiness and love than many people hope to accumulate in a lifetime. He thanks his mother. 'I know that you must be sitting there unbelievingly, ever ready to take on the worries of your children.'

Turning to his wife, he thanks her for standing by him through difficult professional and then personal times. He remembers the day they got married and says that not in his darkest imagination had he considered that one day she would have to live the promise of for better or for worse. He talks frankly about his sorrow in accepting that not only can he no longer safeguard his family but he cannot even care for himself. He tells her that instead of mentioning his courage, people ought to celebrate hers, for enduring eighteen months of suffering by proxy. There is a sense of drama in the room as people listen with bated breath.

Next Tom addresses his daughter. He speaks of his wonder when she was born, of his memory of her first steps, her first words, her first day of school. He tells her how his heart surged with pride each time she simply walked in through the door and greeted him with 'Hi, Daddy!' 'I could never quite believe that I would be blessed with such a wonderful child who fulfilled all my dreams.'

But it is what he says to her last that tears at the heartstrings. 'Get your mother to give you away. I will be watching.' Suddenly, we are all reminded of the grief of a father at losing his daughter. Picturing my baby girl, I close my eyes against the very thought.

Tom uses the final page to thank many other people including his employees, and past employers who gave him a break. I marvel at the way in which he makes each person feel important, obviously one of his many gifts. My attention, fixed on the speech all this time, wavers slightly as I reflect on the sheer calibre of this man. I feel remorseful that the nature of most doctor-patient relationships is such that we come to know barely a fraction of the person behind the patient. Suddenly, I hear the word 'oncologist' mentioned.

'My oncologist is unlikely to be here today,' Tom's friend reads, 'but I want to thank her publicly for the dignity she gave back to me. Oddly enough, it was my last encounter with her that made me see this.'

I imagine a depleted and breathless Tom in his final week of life, remembering to add this in, and my throat constricts with grief and gratitude. Ivana turns to find me in the crowd. I sink back into my seat.

The service ends with a prayer. As the crowd flocks outdoors, I walk up for a closer look at the photograph of Tom. I stand in front of it and hope that he can hear me say thank you for the touching and most unexpected tribute that he thought to pay me. Now that I am closer, I can also read the writing attached to the photograph. It is an excerpt from *Desiderata*, a poem Tom once recited from memory in clinic on a particularly miserable day for him. I remember Tom saying, as if he is seated before me, 'And whatever your labours and aspirations, in the noisy confusion of life, keep peace with your soul. With all its sham, drudgery and broken dreams, it is still a beautiful world. Be cheerful. Strive to be happy.'

I walk out into the sunshine, consoled and inspired.

21

◇

You have helped me decide

It is late at night. My daughter, just past her first birthday, is lying in a hospital crib. Trying to sleep amidst a variety of tubes and machines, she appears a small and desolate figure. The lights are turned off, the only illumination coming from a machine that traces her fast pulse rate and low oxygen levels. Her little frame is rattled by continual coughing, interrupted only when she vomits. She has not eaten in days. When she is too exhausted to protest, she will allow the nurse to coax a few spoonfuls of diluted juice into her mouth before she turns her face away listlessly. She is so tired that she doesn't seem to care who sits in the room beside her, although I have not moved further than the door in the days she has been here.

Both her arms are heavily bandaged and splinted. The nurses say that she deliberately pulls out the nasogastric tube that they have replaced five times in order to give her some feeds, that the only solution is to bandage her arms. I have been there each time the tube fell out – it has been due to the violence of her coughing and not a deliberate act on my daughter's part. I can't help feeling aggrieved at their insinuation. The past twenty-four hours have been particularly trying. The coughing makes her cry with discomfort. The painkillers put her to sleep. The sedation makes it hard to feed her. The lack of feeding causes ongoing weight loss. When you weigh only eight kilograms to begin with, the threshold for anxiety increases. I have stayed awake with her the entire night, tossing on the mattress beside her, wishing that I could inherit her illness because at least I could try to understand my suffering. She can only search my face, whimper, and then return to bed, her eyes glazed, her body exhausted.

The paediatrician says it is only a virus but we don't know yet whether there is anything more to explain her severe symptoms. She deteriorated quickly, within a few days. She should have been in hospital at least twenty-four hours ago. Parents who are doctors tend to fall into two categories. Behind every ailment that their child suffers, there lurks either an incurable cancer or something that needs only a healthy dose of nonchalance to eradicate. I fall into the latter category, arguably equally harmful to a child's well-being as assuming that everything is cancer until proven otherwise. But in doing the work I do, I think it a tremendous disservice to my cancer patients to equate their real and lifelong battles with our thankfully minor colds and coughs that have in the main followed the expected short time course.

However, becoming battle-hardened can sometimes have unintended consequences too, as I now realise. Before the day she was admitted, my daughter had been sick for several days, the last two with a high temperature. She was refusing to eat and drink and went from crying plaintively to becoming quiet, a sign I should have heeded. I called the local emergency department twice and spoke to experienced specialists who I have known and trusted my entire medical career. They said what doctors always say: 'If you are worried, bring her in.' I was worried but I didn't know whether my worry ought to cross the threshold of bothering my overworked colleagues. So I decided to wait until the morning.

My husband slept soundly, suffering from pneumonia and never having been so sick in his adult life. He had just enough energy to look after his own needs before falling back into bed. I did not even think of asking him for his opinion, although he routinely deals with sick children. In retrospect, I have no adequate explanation except my clouded judgement for keeping her at home when she ought to have been in an emergency bay. I do know that if any of my patients had described themselves as so sick, I would have personally ensured that an ambulance picked them up and ferried them to the nearest hospital.

Predictably, the next morning my daughter was worse. We took one look at her, bundled her up in the car and rushed to hospital. If ever there has been a 'guilt trip' in my life, it was this drive to the hospital, where I kept glancing back to make sure that the result of my folly would not worsen in the time it took us to get there. Stopped at a set of lights, I remember thinking how quick doctors are to blame patients for not coming in to hospital, for waiting until they are irredeemably sick. The average patient may be forgiven for not appreciating the seriousness of his symptoms, but what was a doctor's excuse?

Thankfully, she was assessed rapidly and admitted to the children's ward, where she has now been for the past few days. The paediatrician says 'it's behaving like a virus'. He says its effects are 'impressive', that her virus is an 'unknown', that he doesn't 'think there is anything else going on but it would be nice to be sure'. He says that 'sometimes they take a turn for the worse before they improve', that he will be worried 'if things don't look up soon', but right now he is 'feeling comfortable' about the situation.

I use the same phrases on my patients, but suddenly the words seem jarring, even terrifying, in their uncertainty. What they are definitely not is reassuring, these words clothed in caveats. How can it be that even he, a specialist, doesn't know what is ailing my child? The best of medicine defeated, again, by a virus. I accept the principle that finding one culprit organism among the countless viruses that inhabit the air around us is difficult, but the reality is daunting. I am struck by a raw fear because there is no knowing, just waiting.

He tells me about the other tests we could do. 'Only if you must,' I say, hoping he will hear the pleading in my voice. I can't believe how close I am to asking him if I can have those blood tests instead. It is only the thought that he will think me weird and will force me home to sleep that stops me.

Uncertainty has dominated my life in the past few days. I have seen my three-year-old son only occasionally as I pour all my instincts into protecting his tiny, sick sister from real and imagined assaults. The doctors and nurses have delivered care par excellence, but I have realised that even the most resilient of individuals, when placed in the role of parent to a sick child, sheds a part of that resilience to replace it with a thin, very sensitive layer of skin.

The young graduate nurse, with deep blue eyes and blonde curls, says, 'If there is nothing else you want, I am going on my break.' There is in fact nothing else I want but I instinctively withdraw from the steely tone of her voice. Is she implying that I have been a demanding relative, the bane of every nurse? Or is it just a statement meant to inform me of her whereabouts? Why did she say it now, on the day her patient looks at her worst?

My daughter's blood count is marginally abnormal. Her doctor says lightly, 'It doesn't worry me.' But it worries me! I want to shout. It worries me a lot and I want it to worry you, because if you don't worry about *it*, you might forget to worry about *her*.

The pathology nurses come to attack in pairs. 'Do you want to hold her down?' one asks.

'No. I want to be out of the room when you do it.'

'Oh.'

How unhelpful of you, her voice accuses.

'I am sorry,' I feel compelled to say.

There is no response. They are too busy coaxing her collapsed veins. They can't find one and call for reinforcement.

I wander back through the door. 'Do you have children?' I ask the nurse who sounded displeased.

'No, I don't.'

Her answer is my petty vindication. I know that I am not the first mother who refuses to see her child being hurt, however well-intentioned the reason for the pain.

Tonight an older nurse is on duty. She came in earlier and wrapped the baby securely, like we used to swaddle her when she was a newborn. She stroked her head and just stood there, watching her breathing settle as she fell asleep.

'She is a pretty one,' she says, smiling.

There could be no higher form of praise for me.

'How are you doing?' she later asks as she makes my bed against my protests.

'Okay, thank you,' I lie. She does not need two patients in the room.

'Try to get some sleep,' she responds kindly.

'Yes.' My sleep has vanished in a fog of worry and guilt. It will return only with my daughter's health.

The phone rings. It is my parents, their voices weighed with concern. 'Will she be okay?'

'Of course,' I say lightly. 'It's just a virus that needs to run its course.'

'She does look rather sick,' my father observes. He is the contemplative scientist, not prone to exaggeration.

I force myself to respond, 'She will be just fine. We will be home in no time and she will be running around as usual.'

I hang up, my uncertainty multiplied. The nurse is still there. 'You know, dear, I have been a paediatric nurse for thirty years. I have held the sickest children imaginable. But when my infant daughter got sick, nothing compared. The dread was awful. So I just wanted to say I am a mother too. I know how you must feel. But you know what, she will be okay.'

Under cover of darkness, I cry at this spontaneous gesture of humanity. Everyone else, from the cleaner to the paediatrician, has been polite and efficient. My questions have been answered and my doubts addressed. I have never run out of fresh towels or a cool drink and the call bell has always been answered promptly. But it is not until this nurse spoke that I realise what I have been longing for is a show of compassion – for someone to say, it is okay to fret, experience guilt and believe that this is an unmitigated disaster, even if it is clearly not. And for someone to just say aloud, 'I know she will be okay.' For someone to give me permission to discard the mantle of being a doctor and behave like a mother. I feel relieved.

When the nurse leaves, I am unable to sleep, so I walk out of the room to fetch a drink. It is close to ten p.m. Standing at the nurses' desk I see one of my closest friends. 'It's late, I know. I promise I won't stay long.'

My heart soars at this completely unexpected visit. She gives me a hug and tiptoes into the room to see my daughter, who is asleep.

Back in the corridor, she reaches into her bag, and takes out a brown paper bag, which I instantly recognise! In it are two sandwiches from my favourite Vietnamese bakery in a faraway suburb. As medical students on an hour-long drive to our obstetric rotation, we used to be the bakery's first customers. It was a ritual that I particularly enjoyed and she tolerated, my fondness for the sandwich far exceeding her temptation to complain about the daily diversion. I used to say that getting the sandwiches made up for the tedium of waiting for a woman to go into labour.

'I thought you might need these,' she grins, shaking her head at the memory.

I am speechless at her thoughtfulness. After another peek at my daughter, she hurries out under the strict gaze of the staff and I sit alone, devouring the sandwiches, which are as tasty as I remember them. I am comforted by this relic of old times and buoyed by the random act of kindness.

Feeling reassured in mind and full in stomach, I resume my seat outside my daughter's room until I am ready to sleep. A doctor in scrubs knocks confidently at the room next door. At this late hour, he would have to be a surgeon.

'Hey there!' his voice booms. 'I just dropped by to see how you are.'

The patient in that room is an adult who returned from theatre today. I saw him slowly edging towards the bathroom earlier.

'Did you get it all?' he asks.

I go inside, not wanting to listen in, but the doors are thin and the voices loud.

'Ah, it was a good result.'

Watch out, that is not a definitive answer, I say in my own unheard exchange with the patient.

'So it's all clear then?'

'We got most of it and some lymph nodes.'

The subtext is that there was other tumour tissue that was not possible to remove.

'That's great then, yeah? I am okay!'

'Yeah, I am pretty happy with how the surgery went.'

'That's great! If you are happy with the result, so am I!'

Listen carefully, I implore. He is saying it was a good surgical result. That means the surgery achieved what he expected, not necessarily what you were expecting.

'Okay, a few more days and we will get you home.'

'Thanks, doctor!'

'Sure.'

I observe that there is nothing in the surgeon's tone that signals a hint of doubt or caution.

The patient makes a phone call. 'Darling, I just wanted to let you know the surgeon sounded really positive. I should be home in the next few days.' After a pause, he says, 'I told you there was nothing to worry about!'

I groan at this prelude to the patient seeing an oncologist. I can predict the next conversation:

'But my surgeon was really happy.'

'He took out what he could but you will need chemotherapy for the tumour left behind.'

'But he said the operation went well. I thought the tumour was gone.'

'I'm afraid not all of it is gone. This is the reason you are here to see me today.'

'Oh.'

Tonight's exchange will probably never be any of my business, but late at night, it brings home two messages. One, how patients hang on our every word, but especially the positive ones. Which makes it all the more important to ensure that the bad news gets in too, tactfully and considerately. And two, that compared to the uncertainty this man faces, mine is innocuous. Though I am not to know it tonight, it takes just another two days for my daughter to get better. When she eagerly reaches out for her cornflakes, I celebrate. A few hours after that, we are home-bound. It was only a virus: there is no follow-up appointment to keep, no blood tests to repeat and no scans to queue up for in a week or two. It is the outcome every one of my patients would happily trade their circumstances for.

My sleepless, preoccupied mind wanders to my son, who has missed us greatly. This evening, he enquired after his sister before asking conversationally, 'Mama, was her doctor good?' After being slightly taken aback by his comment, it dawned on me that he has probably heard it many times in his parents' conversations. I reassured him that everyone had been good, but did not add that I had now had the opportunity to observe the makings of a good doctor from a very important point of view – that of the patient. It is a view that like all doctors, I don't take into account as often as I should.

With my daughter safely back home, I return to work. Today, I am accompanied by a keen medical student about to graduate and start her internship. She has taken a day out of her term break to follow me around. The hospital being temporarily emptied of her colleagues, she has wisely calculated this as an apt time to attract the full attention of a consultant.

'I have been thinking about doing oncology for some time,' she explains. 'I just want to sit in and see what it's really like.'

I readily agree, even feeling excited by the prospect. Modern medical students have far too many parallel interests to even make it to their scheduled classes, let alone seek out additional engagement. Out of the last batch of students, one was too busy making his first music record. Another was preoccupied with a church retreat and a third confessed to just wanting to be done with his studies and go backpacking. The common refrain one hears these days is, 'Where are the medical students when you need them?' not, 'I have a student who is interested in what I do!'

I start the day feeling important but also slightly nervous at the responsibility bestowed upon me. Medical students and young residents are an impressionable lot – this could be a make or break occasion for her. Stories of how a single experience or conversation changed the life course of a doctor are commonplace. My friend was bent on doing obstetrics until the consultant she admired got sued for delivering a baby who was later diagnosed with cerebral palsy. The case took years to settle but my friend's reaction was instant: 'I am not putting my family through that stress.' Another friend always saw herself as a gastroenterologist until she spent a rotation in neurosurgery. She was converted by the finesse of the surgeon who operated on a bleeding cerebral aneurysm and saved a man's life. She applied to enter surgical training the next day.

The morning begins in outpatients. Irma is the first in line. Since beating the odds in surviving an aggressive bile duct tumour, she is determined to let nothing else get in her way. When I call out her name, she practically runs to greet me. In the office, she plants a kiss on both my cheeks, her eyes shining in genuine delight. I have always admired her capacity to do this at every three-monthly visit, when she has no idea whether or not the results to be revealed in the next few minutes will grant her another reprieve.

'How are you, darling? How are the children?'

The medical student warily regards the overfamiliarity.

'Irma, this is Sheila, she's a medical student. Is it okay if she sits in?'

'Of course, darling!' she beams. 'We all got to learn somewhere!'

We walk through the usual questions, which she answers in her typical fashion. She feels better than ever, she has no symptoms and she is walking along the beach every day, grateful to be alive. I tell her that her results look pristine. She responds by saying she knew all along that she would beat the disease that threatened to end her happy life prematurely. We decide when to schedule her next appointment. Then, out of her bag, she carefully extracts a very large and intricately decorated cake. The student can't contain her gasp at the sophisticated artistry.

'This is for you, darling. It's chocolate this time.'

Although this is Irma's usual ritual, this time I am embarrassed because of the presence of the student.

'Irma is renowned for her cakes,' I say by way of explanation. 'She keeps us all well fed!'

Irma also turns to the student. 'I don't have any words to tell you what she did for me when I was down. The other doctors gave me three months to live, but she took care of me.'

I have always found Irma's enduring gratitude to be touching, although a little misplaced. I have continually told her that she fought her disease, not I, but have come to accept that what she remembers from our very first consultation is my willingness to listen. She has long deleted from her memory my own doubts about her prognosis and her ability to withstand toxic treatment.

As Irma shuts the door behind her, Sheila shakes her head. 'Oh my God, that's wonderful! You must feel so good!'

I quietly think to myself how there is no one else like Irma on my list of patients; that in fact, she defies every stereotype of the cancer patient in remission by being bullishly optimistic to the point of being nonchalant.

'She is nice and her cakes are spectacular!' I say, before calling in the next patient.

I laugh out loud when I see the next name. It is Mrs Milic on her six-monthly visit. Mrs Milic is a delightful Bosnian lady in her eighties. When I met her, she had been on chemotherapy tablets for nearly two years for a low-grade cancer.

'The chemotherapy is a nuisance,' she said. 'And it is stopping me from getting my uterine prolapse repaired because no surgeon will touch me.' Her cancer seemed at bay and I made the decision to stop the troublesome treatment.

'I don't know whether the cancer will come back but I think it's okay to try to come off the tablets and keep you under observation.'

There was not a moment's hesitation in her answer. 'I have been waiting for someone to say this ever since I started them!'

To my relief, the cancer has not grown, the surgeon has repaired her troublesome prolapse, and she is happily carrying on the duties of being the matriarch of her large family. Last year, she decided one appointment every six months was all she could find time for.

Since then, twice a year, Mrs Milic brings a gift for my two children. In summer she uses her well-honed skills to sew them a dress or a shirt; in winter, she knits them each a hat and a scarf. The clothes are immaculately prepared and I have visions of her spending the six months between appointments creating her next pieces. But she brushes away my concerns and reassures me with her toothless grin that she sewed the latest pieces over the weekend between preparing the family feast.

'I don't know whether your son is about to join the circus, doc,' her son simultaneously guffaws and groans. 'I tell her to at least run the colour scheme by us but she won't have any of it!'

As he shields his eyes in mock horror, she proudly holds up a shirt for display. It is fire-engine red, with black and white electric-shock lines running down its entire length. The sharp button-down collar is restrained by glinting black buttons and the sleeves are smartly folded back and held in place by fashionable gold tabs. The overall result is audacious but inexplicably endearing.

'Nothing wrong with them colours! Just 'cos your own son won't wear them. Some people, they like bright colours,' Mrs Milic scolds her sixty-year-old son lovingly.

Focusing on the fine workmanship and reflecting on the dying art of making one's own clothes, I tell Mrs Milic, 'Red is my favourite colour. This is beautiful.'

I steal a sly look at Sheila as I say this, realising that her estimation of my taste must have taken a serious plunge.

Mrs Milic beams. 'Next time I make you another one, different colour. I like you.'

'Mum, what has she done wrong?' her son laughs. 'By the way, do you want to know your blood results?'

Mrs Milic shrugs. 'I feel good. No need blood tests.'

'The tests are indeed good. Maybe we will stop doing them unless they are necessary.'

'I make you winter hat next time.'

'Mrs Milic, you do enough for me. Please don't trouble yourself anymore.'

She leaves the room with loud and good-natured denials about taking any trouble. I fold back my son's red shirt and a prettily embroidered pink frock for my daughter and tuck the gift bag under my desk.

'Do all your patients bring you stuff?' asks Sheila, convinced that my job consists of giving good news and receiving presents and adulation.

'No. Most of my patients are too sick, preoccupied or unhappy,' I answer truthfully.

'It doesn't seem like it today,' she smiles, refusing to be discouraged.

She soon sees what I mean, though. Mr Peterson has progressive mesothelioma which did not respond to chemotherapy. Almost as devastatingly, the chemotherapy gave him months of ringing in the ears before he turned deaf. Although I was careful to mention this uncommon but well-known side effect to him, I did not expect him to suffer from it. No one will say it outright but his entire family holds me silently responsible for the disaster. His daughter, a nurse, scowls at me each time he adjusts his hearing aid. Today, he has come to seek my permission to travel to the United States for three months: 'I am off treatment anyway and it's something I have always wanted to do.'

Alarm bells ring inside my head. I have had frank discussions with him before about his limited life expectancy. The mesothelioma has progressed and I suspect he does not have long to live. I am concerned about his ability to tolerate the long flight to Arizona, but even more about the likelihood of his becoming progressively ill and requiring specialised medical care. His insurance will not cover him, leaving him with a potentially huge bill.

'So what do you think?'

He looks uncomfortable; I think he will need oxygen soon, and ongoing adjustment to his pain medications. I know that the family views my role as the spoiler and I am keen to make something right for him, but I am also obliged to tell the truth.

'I wish I could say yes, but my fear is that if you were to fall ill in Arizona, you would get stuck and not be able to return home. America is also a very expensive place to get sick, Mr Peterson.'

'But they have great care over there,' his daughter interrupts. This is not the first time she has suggested that her father has been short-changed by me, although despite my encouragement, she has steadfastly declined to take her father for a second opinion.

'I agree that they have cutting-edge technology and access to the newest drugs and I am sure you could find a very good oncologist if you needed one. I could look someone up for you.'

'But I want to travel around when I am there.'

'Mr Peterson, I am sorry but I don't think that's wise.' I quietly grimace at his lack of appreciation for his own incapacity.

'But it's up to us as a family to decide,' his daughter barks back.

I hold my tongue and continue to address her father. 'I will do whatever I can to help. If you want to travel, I will make sure you have all the necessary paperwork from this end.'

He slowly turns a pen around in his hand. 'I need to think about it. I am going to go home and think about it.'

I am disappointed that he doesn't detect the urgency in my voice or seize the opportunity to wonder why I am so concerned. However, I feel as if I have fulfilled my role of his advisor. I offer to see him in four weeks but he wants the appointment for much later to fit in a possible trip.

After he leaves, Sheila observes, '*They* seemed a bit unhappy.'

The next patient we see has liver secondaries. His jaundiced skin glows a fluorescent yellow. With bony hands and gnarled fingers, he withdraws a newspaper cut-out from his pocket. The article documents the successful liver transplant of Apple's CEO, Steve Jobs, whose battle with cancer is said to be over.

'Doc, nobody never told me I could get a liver transplant,' he says, a touch miffed.

I groan quietly. Celebrities with cancer can raise awareness but many patients do just what Tony is doing. They wonder why their case is different.

'Tony, liver transplants are not usually performed for cancer.'

'But they gave this guy one.'

'Tony, it's not standard procedure. His case must be exceptional.'

'Yeah, he is rich.'

'That he is, Tony,' I am forced to agree. 'But it's not lack of money that is holding you back from a liver transplant.'

He grumbles under his breath, not entirely convinced. I am sorry that he came across the article. Steve Jobs' doctors must seem even more of a world away for this poor man, who is reliant on a government pension to buy his groceries.

The two women who follow Tony are both five years past their breast cancer diagnosis. Both are still young – in their forties – and so their risk of a late relapse is still significant. Sharing in their relief to have come so far, I touch on the importance of remaining vigilant without being over-anxious. I feel let off when, overcome by relief, neither questions how to make this possible. For I don't know. I don't know that if I was struck by cancer, I could take my own advice of getting on with life. It sounds good and it sounds logical, but as the years pass, I meet few patients able to live by what their doctor preaches.

As we snatch a break to have a drink, Sheila says to me, 'It's hard work, isn't it?'

I smile. 'I think all patient care is, don't you?'

'Your job seems harder.'

Her words prove prophetic. Mr Coleman is sixty but looks twenty years older. His gait, aided by permanent crutches, is as slow as it is painful. When he broke his hip on Christmas Eve, the attending orthopaedic surgeon described the result as 'mangled'. No amount of surgery, radiation therapy or physiotherapy has managed to solve the problem. His much younger wife, whom I initially mistook for his daughter, looks up as I call his name. Leaving him to crawl at his own pace into my office, she covers the short distance in a few long strides. The contrast between the couple is stark.

She quickly enters the room and, before I have had a chance

to say anything, she whispers conspiratorially, 'I can't do this! You must talk to him about going somewhere.'

Sheila looks back and forth between us. I only have time to mutter, 'He has metastatic colon cancer and is declining rapidly,' before he is within earshot.

'Hi, Mr Coleman,' I greet him. 'How are things?'

'Ah, not good,' he sighs and yelps as he disengages himself stiffly from his crutches.

I decide to involve Sheila in the conversation with the obliging man. Every medical student knows the 'pain questions' verbatim.

'Mr Coleman, last time we met, you had a lot of pain. Do you mind if I get Sheila to ask you a few questions about your pain?'

'No, no. Not at all.'

Sheila springs out of her chair eagerly. 'Mr Coleman, where is your pain?'

'Here, love.' He jabs at his bad hip and lower back. 'But actually all over.'

'Does it go anywhere? Oh, I guess you just told me. Does anything make it better?'

'No. Hard to tell.'

'Does anything make it worse?'

'Hard to say when you are always in pain.'

I can see Sheila is a little nonplussed at his answers, which do not follow the neat pattern she has been taught. And if she has been hoping for a eureka moment, it is not going to come from her final question, which figures high on my list of pointless medical questions. She asks it with immense honesty and hope: 'Mr Coleman, if ten is the worst pain you have ever had, and one is, like, minor pain, how would you rate your pain on a scale of one to ten?'

As I watch his face contort in an expression very familiar

to me and which prompts his wife to reach into her bag for some morphine, I can't help but be reminded of just how frustrating and useless I found the question when I was admitted to hospital in premature labour. It was the most uncomfortable pain I had ever experienced but was it because I was not resilient enough or was it truly meant to be so painful? How seriously would someone take my self-rated pain, especially when my mind was clouded by the symptom? More importantly, would the rating make the difference between someone just stroking my hand or injecting me with a strong painkiller, which is what I was desperate for?

The student midwife's face floated in and out before mine as I clutched my pregnant abdomen. 'I am in a lot of pain,' I said in a tearful voice.

'How would you rate it on a scale of one to ten?'

'Five,' I replied, thinking it would convey a degree of seriousness without seeming self-indulgent.

'Oh, so it's not too bad.'

My heart sank at the lost opportunity. I ended up not receiving any pain relief and kicked myself for the mistake. Ever since, I don't ask this question of my patients.

'Mr Coleman, do you think you can rate your pain?' Sheila prompts.

'Eleven out of ten, love.'

'Oh.'

I take over. 'You have had bad pain for months. You are on nearly four hundred milligrams of morphine a day. We need to switch drugs.'

'Okay, I trust you.'

I glance at his wife before focusing my attention on him. 'Do you remember we talked about admitting you to hospice for better pain management? I really feel that you need to be closely monitored by a pain doctor, Mr Coleman, and I think we can get this under control.'

'Hmm . . . You can't do it at home?'

'The drugs I want to try need very close supervision, although once you are established on them, a nurse can visit you at home.'

'George, come on. You have to try it. This could make all the difference.' His wife looks hopeful.

He scratches his chin, as if seriously considering the matter, but then says what he has done each time: 'I just don't think I want to go to hospice.'

'George is afraid that once he goes to hospice, that's it.' She sighs, looking away.

Regarding him, I can see why he is afraid. There is a good chance that once he sinks into the comfort of hospice, he will relax and let go. His scans also tell a story of disease ready to deteriorate into its terminal stages without further warning. His refusal to enter hospice is a reflection of his grasp on life, however tenuous; he does not want to cede this last vestige of control to others.

'Not every one goes to hospice to die,' I say gently. 'There are patients like you who need difficult symptoms managed before they go back home.'

'It's not like they are just going to keep you there forever against your wishes, George,' his wife urges.

Her last statement has the unintended effect of making me deeply uncomfortable. My mind flies back to a patient who desperately wanted to die at home. But seemingly everything and everyone conspired against his plan because we saw that his care needs were far too complex. He never understood or accepted our decision, which contributed to significant depression at the end of his life. But his wife did not want him home, petrified that she would err in her care. His elderly parents felt most secure when he was in our care and so it came to be that his plea was crowded out by the consensus decision. It may have been the right practical decision but I still grapple with the moral dimensions of it.

'Mr Coleman, you are right in thinking that sometimes people intend to leave hospice but don't manage to because their care needs increase.'

'See, I told you so,' he asserts to his wife.

His wife shrugs. She knows her husband is going to be one of those patients but she wants him in hospice nonetheless.

'I still think that we can do better with your pain if you would just let us try in hospice.'

'I will think about it, doctor. I am just not keen on hospice.'

His wife's frustration bursts its dam. 'George, you know you are going to have to think about other people in this, how it impacts on them. Other people are involved too.'

She stops abruptly. I feel sorry for her. She has used up all her fortitude not to substitute 'I' for 'other people'. Her compassion for him is obvious but it has been an arduous journey since he broke his hip ten months ago. Lately, he has become so dependent that she has been forced to leave work and accept a meagre carer's pension in place of her comfortable salary. She spends all day and night tending to a man who is no longer the person she married. She has said to me before, 'He is on so many drugs that he can't really talk meaningfully. If he was comfortable, I could accept it. But it kills me to see him suffering like this and not being able to do anything.'

He only half hears her through the haze of drugs and pain. Or perhaps he just doesn't know what to say because he has heard it all before. They leave the room, the tentative hope for a resolution again firmly replaced by tension.

'What do you think will happen to him?'

'He will die a miserable death at home and his wife will be sad but very relieved,' I say, not bothering to mince my words.

Sheila draws her breath at my inelegant conclusion. She has yet to learn that sometimes detachment is the only possible retreat from a testing encounter.

We see a further smattering of patients, some routine reviews and others with relatively minor issues related to ongoing chemotherapy. I dispense with them quickly, glad for the respite.

'I am done seeing patients here,' I say. 'There is some dictation and paperwork left but you may go.'

'Is that it for you?'

'No, I have a new consult on the ward. The poor guy came in with a clot in his leg and the medical team found a lung cancer.'

'Can I come?'

I am surprised. I thought she would have had enough.

'It will be more of the same, I am afraid,' I say, nevertheless impressed by her tenacity.

'I have never seen someone give a new diagnosis of cancer to a patient. If you don't mind, I would love to see how you do it.'

Of all the interactions with patients, relating a new diagnosis is one of the hardest and the one that never becomes routine. It is the first fall of the oncologist's gavel in a patient's life. It will sound many more times but never with the same gravity. This is the date and this is the conversation that becomes etched in patients' memories for the remainder of their lives.

'When was your cancer diagnosed?' I recently asked a patient as I distractedly looked through his thick file in order to fill out his insurance forms.

'The 26th of June 2006,' he said automatically, as if reciting his birthday. Almost every subsequent detail he recalled was inexact but not the date he was told he had cancer.

The new consult is a young man and I would much prefer to handle him alone, but I feel obliged to teach the rare student who really wants to be taught.

'Sure. Do you want a ride to the hospital?'

'Okay!' she responds happily.

During the short trip to the hospital, she talks about her experience in medicine so far.

'My problem is that I like almost everything. So I really have to think about what to do.' The inevitable follows: 'Did you always want to be an oncologist?'

'I knew very early that I was cut out to be a physician but exactly what sort took time to work out.'

'So how did you decide, because that's my fear. What if I decide on the wrong thing?'

'You will know, trust me.'

I suppress a grin at sounding like an agony aunt counselling a worried teenager about finding the right life partner. I am on the verge of telling her my story but I draw back, conscious that it might sound lame to someone very bright, who expects more logical decision-making.

'I hope so. It must be nice to know your place.'

The mistaken perception of others can sometimes be a comfort in its own way. She doesn't know how many times I come home questioning what I do. She has not heard the troubling questions I ask myself about my role, supposedly that of a healer, but too often trumped by fate or misfortune as I am forced to look on, the very opposite of a dispassionate observer.

I park the car and enter through the emergency department. The first person I run into is Harry, an orderly who has been there for as long as I can remember. Harry was diagnosed with colon cancer a few years ago and took many months to recover. I only heard the news on the grapevine and when he made his improbable return to work, I decided not to remind him of his ordeal but told him that I had missed him. We have never spoken of his cancer, but he innocently assumes that, being an oncologist, I must know all about his battle and this is how we have developed an unspoken bond.

'Hey, doc!' he beams. 'Busy at work?'

Harry's welcome feels like a favourite pair of jeans.

Sheila and I enter the general medical ward and head straight for the room of Mr Naeem Uddin. The room is separated by curtains into three cubicles. The curtains are drawn closed around the middle cubicle but we can see Mr Uddin through the window. We walk into his space and I introduce us. He is seated at his table, leafing through a motoring magazine. He is in his early forties and at first glance looks well. His small cubicle is neatly arranged. A vase of flowers sits atop a large box of chocolates. An information booklet lies face down on the table. It is the only giveaway that he may have cancer.

'Mr Uddin, your physicians have asked me to come around and talk to you about your diagnosis and where to go from here. Were you expecting me?'

'Yes, doctor.'

'Mr Uddin, I understand that you came into hospital with a spontaneous blood clot in your leg and since then, your doctors have picked up a lung cancer.'

'Yes.'

Just at this moment, the curtains to the cubicle next door swing open and shut and the booming but genial voice of a colleague interrupts my exchange with Mr Uddin.

'Hello there, Lizzie!' he greets his patient. 'How are you doing today?'

'Hi, doctor.' Lizzie sounds about eighteen.

What follows is an extraordinary juxtaposition of consultations involving Lizzie and her doctor and Mr Uddin and myself, both within clear earshot of one another.

'Lizzie, the tests came back. You have a simple urinary tract infection,' he says.

'Oh, that's it? Nothing more serious than that?'

'Mr Uddin, the radiologist also suspects that your adrenal glands might be abnormal. This means the cancer has spread outside the lung.'

'So this is very serious, doctor.'

'Young women are particularly prone to getting these infections. A course of antibiotics should get you better in no time. And you need to drink plenty of water.'

'Mr Uddin, you need another scan. You are young; we want to remove the cancer if possible.'

'And if it's not operable?'

'Then you will need chemotherapy.'

'I hate antibiotics. They mess with my skin. How many do I need?'

'Only for two more days.'

'I hear chemotherapy makes you very sick. Will it go for long?'

'A few months.'

'My mum said to ask if these infections can cause long-term damage.'

'Not if they are infrequent and promptly treated, like yours is. The scan shows your kidneys are just fine.'

'My wife said to ask if there is a cure for this kind of cancer.'

'I am afraid there is no guarantee of a cure even if we manage to remove the cancer.'

'Doctor, can I go home soon? I miss home.'

'Sure, Lizzie. I think we can let you go tomorrow. You will be fine by Wednesday.'

'Doctor, can you keep me here till all the tests are done? It will be hard for my wife to drive me around and my leg is still very painful.'

'Sure. I think you should stay for as long as necessary and we will try to expedite all the tests and even get started on treatment.'

'That's great! Thanks for fixing me!'

'No problems, Lizzie. You take care now,' he says lightly, as he draws back the curtains.

'Doctor, I have a few more questions. Please let me have a drink of water and wait for my head to settle down.'

'There is no rush. Why don't we step out for a second?'

'Mum, I am coming home! Doctors are so cool! He has completely fixed me!' Lizzie says. I have stepped outside my patient's curtain and can see her madly texting with one hand as she cradles the hospital phone between her ear and neck.

I watch the jaunty steps of my colleague carry him into another room, probably to deliver another neat parcel of good news to an eager and grateful patient.

Just then, for good measure, the surgeon pops into the third cubicle. In the years that I have known him, I have never seen him walk. There is a joke that in order to catch him, you need to run the minute you spot him, because he will disappear into the operating theatre in the blink of an eye.

'Hello, Mrs Vo!' he shouts a little too loudly at the delicate Vietnamese lady who is dozing in bed. Mrs Vo nearly falls out of bed.

'Your appendix, gone. Your pneumonia, fixed. It's home for you!'

He prances out of the room, whistling as poor Mrs Vo tries to make sense of who on earth the man was and what he just shouted at her. I calculate that it takes me as much time to introduce myself as it has taken the surgeon to dispense with a patient! Awake now, she spots me and painstakingly reaches for a sign that says, 'I speak Vietnamese.' In spite of the situation, I cannot suppress a laugh behind my file.

But as I return with the medical student to my hapless patient, waiting to unfold bad news like one peels an onion, I am struck by an unforeseen pang of jealousy. I want to have what these other doctors are having. I want to be able to say with a swing of my stethoscope and a gaiety to my tone that somebody is cured. I want to take the credit for banishing a patient's nuisance illness, like a misbehaving appendix or a pesky urinary tract infection. Just once, I want someone to call their family and say I fixed them and said never to worry again. But cancer is unfair not just to patients, but also in some measure to their oncologists.

Sheila watches from a seat in the corner as I handle a series of remarkably well-thought out and mature questions from a man who is still discovering the full implications of having cancer. He assumes the worst-case scenario and asks questions about chemotherapy and its side effects. Satisfied, he moves on to other practicalities like how much time off he will need from his job as a software engineer and whether his wife will need help looking after their two children on the days after chemotherapy when he is feeling sick. He wants to know about my experience with similar patients and whether he has missed out on asking me anything important.

'No, I don't think so, Mr Uddin,' I reassure him. 'I think you have done a very thorough job today.'

'I feel like you can never be too prepared.'

'I can understand that.'

'Doctor, one more thing.'

'Sure.'

'We have all got to die sometime. All I ask is that you are honest with me so that I can prepare my wife and children for whatever is coming. Safeguarding their future is more important to me than getting a few more weeks out of my life.'

His gallant request moves me and reminds me that this is one area where the patient's request always seems more poignant because we do a poor job of granting it. I wonder whether he has had a prior bad experience but instead, summoning my enthusiasm, I say, 'Let's get some treatment started to make you feel better. You are a long way from dying yet.'

'Thank you, doctor, for being so kind.'

Outside, Sheila hovers politely as I finish writing my notes. I can sense from her fidgeting that she is burning with questions. No sooner have I shut the file than she proclaims, 'How can you do this?'

'Do what?' I hear her question at least once or twice a day.

'Do this. Isn't it depressing?' She stops, fearing she has gone too far in her criticism.

'What did you find depressing?'

'All of it!' she answers.

'Even the clothes Mrs Milic made my children?' I say, laughing.

Sheila giggles, relaxing now that I have not taken offence. 'I guess what I am saying is you deal with so much stuff. Isn't it hard?'

'Patients would still get cancer and suffer the same symptoms whether I am an oncologist or not. But if I can help them deal with it in some way, I feel that's a worthy task.'

'That's a good way of looking at it,' she says, nodding appreciatively.

'Have you rotated through other wards?'

'Yes, lots.'

'Did you meet any diabetics?'

'I will never forget the last diabetic patient I interviewed. He was fifty-six years old, with both legs amputated due to gangrene and one arm disabled after a fistula infection. He was on hemodialysis and had spent six out of the last twelve months in hospital. Everyone felt sorry for the poor guy because now he was going blind and would have to be placed in a nursing home. But he was just so nice that even the professors felt sorry for him.'

'And was that an extreme case or did you see others like him?'

'I must say that the renal ward was mostly filled with chronic sufferers who had the most awful complications. Sometimes even they wondered why they were still alive.'

'Have you seen anyone with severe emphysema?'

'All the time. There was a lady who came in four times during my monthly rotation. She was on home oxygen and very fragile. The resident told me to listen to her lungs because she had pneumonia but even sitting up in bed made her gasp. Every admission, she came close to a code blue. Every time we had the same conversation with her: "Thelma, what do you want us to do if you stop breathing?"'

'How long had Thelma been like that?'

'For years, but the last year had been especially terrible. She just wanted it to end.'

'So how are these life-threatening diseases that rob you of any meaningful quality of life any different to having cancer?'

Sheila looks at me with wide open eyes.

'If you put it like that, it's not really, is it? But, just the very word cancer causes dread, whereas renal failure or emphysema you think you can live with.'

'What's in a word?' I muse, as we continue to walk along.

'I think you need to be pretty together to do your kind of work,' she says in an admiring tone.

'Or,' I reply mildly, 'you learn from your patients how to be strong because they are the remarkable ones.'

She falls silent until she asks to be dropped off at the train station so she can make her way home.

'It has been a long day for you. Thank you for coming along.'

Another quick checkout of a career in oncology, I think wryly.

'No, thank you. You have helped me decide that this is what I want to do.'

Childlike, my heart soars.

22

◇

The makings of a good doctor

Among the most memorable days of my life is the one on which I received news that I had been accepted to study medicine. I remember the joy and pride that flowed untrammelled through my family's heart. I felt as if my acceptance into medicine was a confirmation that society was willing to allow me the privilege of making a difference. Many professions perform valuable and generous services but there is something very special about being entrusted with the care of the sick and the vulnerable. I pledged then to work hard and be the best possible doctor.

With this in mind, I asked a medical student recently what defined a good doctor. 'Sure,' he said. 'It's someone who knows what they are doing, who can confidently fix peoples' problems and tell them what's wrong.' As an afterthought he added, 'Oh, and it probably helps if they are nice.' I put the same question to an eighty-year-old neighbour. She responded, 'Darling, to us common people, you are all experts. I like mine because he waits patiently while I struggle with my hearing aid.'

A good doctor recognises that the essence of medical practice lies in its art. It lies in listening, reading between the lines and reaching out. It is recognising that there is more to a disease than its physical symptoms and there is more to a physician than fixing these symptoms. It took me the first few years of being a doctor to realise this, none more so than when I first did oncology.

All too often doctors define themselves by their profession. Having spent a substantial part of my life getting here, being a doctor is a strong part of my own identity. Yet with time, I have become wary of making it my sole identity. The day-to-day contact with my patients has prompted me to define myself in other ways: a loyal friend, a devoted mother or a caring relative. Or connecting with my neighbours and volunteering. Without ever saying it, my patients have taught me to defend life actively against seeming hollow one day when the doctor's sign comes off the door.

One of the most exciting things about being a doctor can also be one of its disadvantages: you never stop learning. And the more you learn and meet truly scintillating individuals, the more tempted you are to climb to greater professional heights. You develop a skewed view of success and it never seems like a good time to get married, have children, take that long-awaited holiday or call your childhood friend. One of the most common conversations I have with my female residents these days is about the best time to have children and how and when to return to medicine.

In my work, I have yet to meet a patient who rues wasted career opportunities, but I do see the busy diplomat who wished he had been at his son's high-school graduation, the mother who was too busy keeping the house clean to spend more time with her children before they left home, and the woman who could find neither time nor money to marry her fiancé until she became too ill to leave her hospital bed. Sometimes all it takes is a glance at the dusty pile of medical journals heaped on my bedside table to reignite my own professional anxieties but I see more clearly now that in a life overflowing with opportunities, you are responsible for the choices you make, and that an unchecked competitive streak is not without consequence.

One of the professional choices I make several times during the day is how to best use my time with patients. Patients wait to see their doctor with anticipation and trepidation but most of all, with hope. They have run through more worst-case scenarios than I could imagine – I don't need to account for their unpaid mortgage, their beloved dog or the blind neighbour whose groceries they have fetched every week for the past ten years.

Early in my career, I felt my primary duty was to impart medical facts. There were other people who were better equipped to handle the social and emotional fallout from cancer. But though the patients seemed accepting enough, my interactions felt incomplete. It bothered me that the confidence a patient showed in me may be limited to my ability to explain the sterile details of his or her cancer and the proposed treatment schedule. But what if I asked the burning question in my mind, 'How are you really doing?' and someone actually chose to respond honestly? Did I have the time or ability to deal with the myriad thoughts and doubts that crisscrossed the mind of every cancer patient?

There was no way to know but try to bring the consultation to a more human level, to actively ask patients about their moods, fears or wishes. I realise now that I have never had cause to regret the approach. And even with the little I sometimes feel able to do, I am touched by my patients' assertion when they say, 'I feel better after talking to you.'

Being mindful of the lives of patients has made me more mindful of their deaths, too. One of my very first patients bled to death. I still remember the impact of witnessing that barbaric death and even now, walking past the room transports me back to that afternoon.

My hands shook as I wrote the death certificate.

My first few losses after this made me sad and introspective, but some years later, especially on busy nights, I found myself certifying deaths as if writing a prescription for an antibiotic. Now, I close the door behind me and spend a still moment taking in the surroundings. I look at greying wedding photographs and pictures pasted on cardboard, depicting regular family events; a profusion of cards, some with a child's wobbly drawing or handwriting; flowers from a well-tended garden; the last music the patient listened to; the last book he read. This moment reminds me that every death robs someone of a child, sibling, parent or partner. Every death closes the book on a life that I barely knew. And I am reminded to not be arrogant before death. A quiet and reflective moment spent in the presence of the dead provides fresh insight into the gift of life.

Despite many advances in oncology, a large proportion of my patients succumb to their disease. I would not have thought it, but one of my most cherished tasks is to call their surviving family. I still approach the task feeling tentative, not knowing whether the relatives will choose to cast blame on the disease or the doctor. This fear sometimes leads me to avoid calling certain families, but I am struck by the surprise and gratitude of grieving relatives for a simple phone call. In all these years, I cannot recall a family that has taken undue advantage of the gesture, but many have said that it has renewed their faith in the medical profession to be remembered in the aftermath of their loved one's demise.

A colleague sets aside time to write notes to relatives. Once, a copy mistakenly arrived on my desk. I did not know the patient but reading the note caused a lump in my throat. In just a few words, the letter celebrated the elderly man and saluted his wife for undertaking the demanding journey of cancer with him. It is hard to overestimate the consolation his words must have brought.

But perhaps the single most important thing that I have learnt from being an oncologist is to be grateful. I am simply grateful for my life and for my health. Many of my patients have incurable cancer. Lately, I have taken to closely observing the trigger that led to their diagnosis. The answers are so benign that they would invite good-humoured disbelief were it not for the patient sitting before me. 'My hand just went to it.' 'My job required a chest X-ray.' 'I turned in bed and just felt a lump.' Many patients were leading a perfectly normal life in the days or weeks before the calamity fell. Their revelations are a sobering reminder of the instant power of disease to change our lives. What I have learnt from my patients is that it often takes the diagnosis of a dire illness for them to re-evaluate their life and place the small things in perspective. 'That poor girl,' an old lady once remarked, 'she looks so sick. I don't mind if you see her first.' I looked at her in admiration. She had a brain full of metastases yet she cared for someone else's welfare.

My patients talk to and about their children more. My patients worry less about money, fame or fashion, and concentrate more on being at peace with themselves and with society at large. They have finally come to understand and despise the trivial issues that we let crowd our lives. Maybe it really is as simple as that. But I never fail to wonder what it is in our make-up that prevents us from appreciating these things earlier. I am grateful for being able to think, talk and walk. Life is good just as it is. And on the days that my own mind needs convincing, I simply stop by at a patient's bedside.

Acknowledgements

Some years ago, when I was a new oncologist and this book was just a kernel of an idea, my brother and I were stuck in airport traffic. My assertion that the remarkable stories I witnessed every day needed to be told was yet to be matched by my confidence in doing them justice. My initial gratitude must go to my brother for his breezy conviction, which made up for my lack of it.

My mother and father have never successfully retired from the task of nurturing my interests and implicitly trusting in the worth of my endeavours: no gesture seems adequate to express how indebted I am to them.

To my husband, Declan, I owe enormous thanks for the onerous task of most often being charged with sifting through incomplete ideas and unfinished drafts, which he fulfilled late at night with interest and goodwill in the times he was not minding our children.

My beloved children, whose most frequent question was, 'Mama, are you being an author again?' were my fondest inspiration and most innocent distraction. Although they are too young to understand now, I hope they will one day recognise the extraordinary privilege I have in being a doctor and why I needed to write about it.

My ideas for a book would have remained just that were it not for the introduction, by way of Ian Hamilton, Robert Fisher and Bob Sessions, to Andrea McNamara, my publisher at Penguin. From our first meeting, Andrea invested in me with exemplary grace, patience and respect, remarkably never running out of ways to improve on the improvements. She is an author's dream come true. Andrea also introduced me to two exceptional editors, Jo Jarrah and Julia Carlomagno, who so enthusiastically and painstakingly polished my work when I found it hard to view it with meaningful objectivity.

I have been fortunate to ride on the wings of support of far too many people around the world. In particular, I thank Swati Jha, Wendy Schmidt, Roger Short, Kwai Lee, John Scarlett, Warren Hastings, Mark Siegler and my colleagues at the MacLean Center, Ramesh Nagappan, Rosemary and Geoffrey Green, Taru Sinha, Geraldine Buckingham, Hanita Gandhi, Leena Narain and Debbie Malina.

It would be remiss of me to not mention my English teacher from Pittsburgh, Wayne Sommerfeld, who taught me the secret of writing with just three words: 'Put me there!' Whenever I was stuck for words, I only had to take my mind back to his invaluable advice.

But I reserve my deepest and most heartfelt gratitude for my patients and their families. Without their remarkable generosity and candour in letting me into their world at its most devastating, there would be no book, but more importantly, I would be a lesser individual, denied the rich perspective that is mine for life.

ALSO BY DR RANJANA SRIVASTAVA

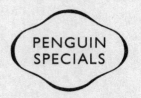

DYING FOR A CHAT

Shortlisted for the 2013 Human Rights Literature Award

Why good communication skills should be considered as important to healthcare as medical breakthroughs.

Medical oncologist Ranjana Srivastava contends that the best medicine begins with a good chat, to guide the decision-making of both doctors and patients. Increasingly, people are unable to properly comprehend the complex treatment choices on offer, or are self-diagnosing and demanding unnecessary or risky procedures. Doctors, in turn, feel unable to deny the requests of patients and their families. Narrow specialisation also means no-one is discussing the overall picture of a patient's health. Srivastava warns that people are suffering – even dying – as a result, and the medical profession should be taking responsibility. In a frank and clear-eyed assessment of an unacknowledged crisis, she makes an impassioned case for healthcare training to incorporate effective communication skills.

'A humane treatise exploring the relationship between doctors and their patients.' *West Australian*